DIAGNOSTIC PICTURE TESTS IN

UROLOGY

N. J. R. George
MD, FRCS

Senior Lecturer and Consultant in Urology
University Hospital of
South Manchester, England

P. Sambrook
FRCR

Consultant Radiologist
University Hospital of
South Manchester, England

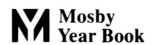

Mosby
Year Book

St. Louis   Baltimore   Boston   Chicago   London   Philadelphia   Sydney   Toronto

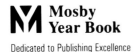

Mosby
Year Book

Dedicated to Publishing Excellence

Mosby–Year Book, Inc.
11830 Westline Drive
St. Louis, MO 63146

ISBN 0-8016-6289-3

English edition first published in 1991 by Wolfe Publishing Ltd,
2–16 Torrington Place, London WC1E 7LT, UK.

Printed in the United Kingdom.

Library of Congress Cataloging-in-Publication Data has been
applied for.

Preface

There can be few branches of medicine that illustrate the rapid evolution of diagnostic techniques as well as the speciality of urological surgery. From 'cutting for stone' to Extra-corporeal Shock Wave Lithotripsy, the art of the nineteenth century has turned into the space age science of the twenty-first; the present-day urologist has inherited a wealth of technical ingenuity undreamed of by his forebears.

Modern diagnostic urology is thus able to call upon a complex blend of symptoms, an assortment of visual and palpable signs and a formidable array of radiological scans, biochemical assays and pathophysiological measurements. This text, therefore, not only illustrates common pathological processes by conventional means, but also explains the nature and drawbacks of available investigations, the rationale for their use and the specific aims of treatment. Some diseases are discussed from a variety of standpoints; other disorders are included because they demonstrate the advantages of a particular line of investigation or the limitation of certain tests. Throughout, the essential and expanding contribution of radiology to urological practice is emphasized in depth.

It is to be hoped that both undergraduate and postgraduate students will benefit from this educational approach, which seeks to replace the tedium of learning 'parrot fashion' by the more rewarding experience of pursuing knowledge by rational analysis and reasoned argument.

Acknowledgements

We gratefully acknowledge the cooperation of the Medical Illustration Department, Withington Hospital, who are responsible for much of the clinical photography in this book. We also thank consultant colleagues and those patients who allowed themselves to be photographed. Mrs Gillian Trimble kindly typed the text.

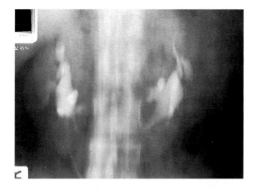

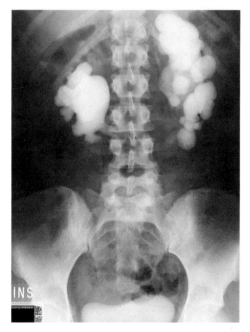

1, 2 IVU examinations of patients **1** and **2** with the same congenital anomaly.

(a) What is the underlying lesion?

(b) What complication does the patient in **2** show?

(c) What other complications occur in this condition?

(d) What unassociated abnormality is present in the left kidney of the patient in **1**?

3

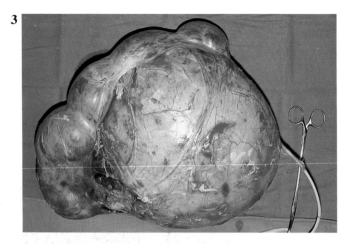

4

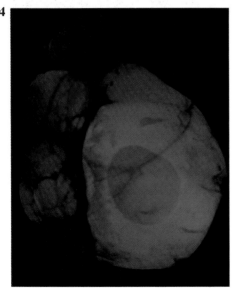

3, 4 (a) What is this congenital disorder?
(b) What is the important feature shown?
(c) What are the characteristic symptoms?
(d) What is the usual treatment?

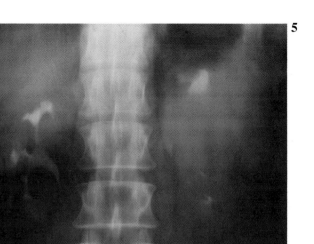

5 (a) What is this lesion?
(b) What are the usual presenting clinical features?
(c) What are less common presentations?
(d) What is the next essential radiological investigation?

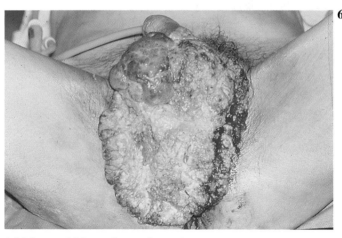

6 Male, aged 76, continuous incontinence.
(a) What is this lesion?
(b) What predisposing factors may influence development?
(c) What is the treatment?
(d) In this case, how may urinary leakage be treated?

7

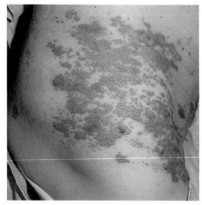

7 Male, 70, metastatic prostatic cancer.
(a) What is this lesion?
(b) What is its significance?
(c) How might this be confusing?
(d) What other enquiry might be made?

8

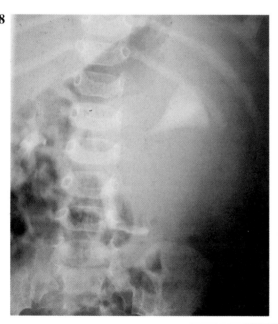

8 (a) What is the abnormality?
(b) What is the usual age of presentation?
(c) What are the usual clinical features?
(d) What is the common site of metastatic spread?

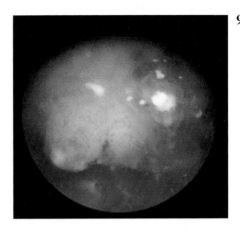

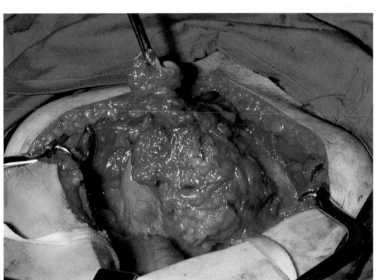

9, 10 Male, aged 72: blood and mucus per urethram.
(a) What is this disorder?
(b) How common is it?
(c) Where does it originate?
(d) What is the primary treatment?

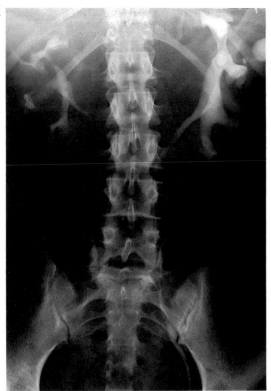

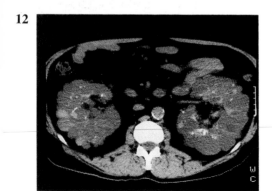

11, 12 (a) What does this IVP show?
(b) What is a more accurate method of imaging this condition?
(c) What is the mode of inheritance?
(d) What are the usual clinical presenting features?

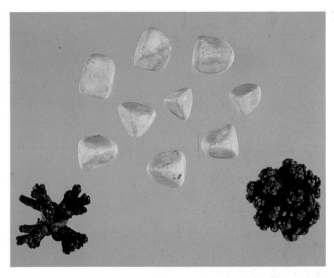

13 Bladder stones.
(a) What is the likely composition of the spiky 'jack stone'?
(b) What may predispose to the multiple chalky stones?
(c) What is the geographical distribution for bladder stone?
(d) What bladder wall defect predisposes to stone formation?

14 (a) What is this bladder disorder seen at laparotomy?
(b) What symptoms are commonly present?
(c) What treatment is effective?
(d) What may happen to renal function?

15

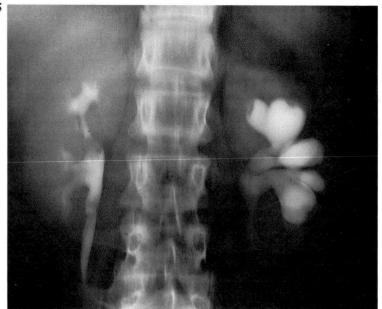

16

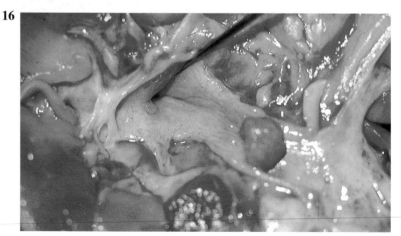

15, 16 X-ray and specimen of right kidney.
(a) What is observed?
(b) What is likely to have been the presenting symptom?
(c) What is the advised treatment?
(d) What regular follow up treatment will be required?

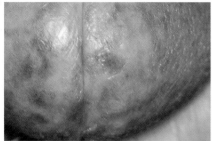

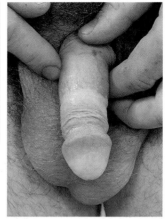

17, 18 (a) What is this condition?
(b) What complications may occur?
(c) What treatment may be offered?

19 (a) What is this lesion?
(b) What is the usual mode of spread?
(c) What histological appearances may be expected?
(d) What is the primary mode of therapy?

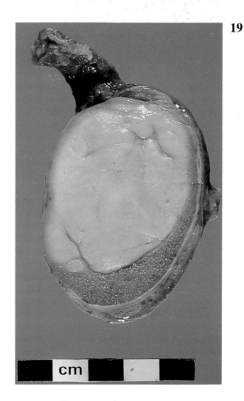

20

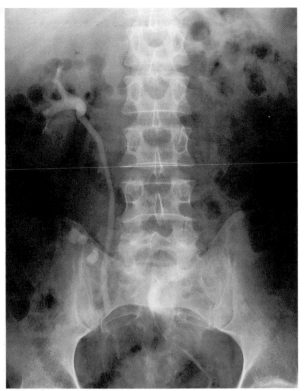

21

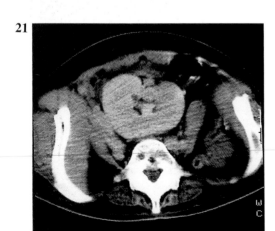

20, 21 These two males show variations of a congenital abnormality.
(a) What is this condition?
(b) How may this present?
(c) From where is the arterial blood supply likely to be taken?

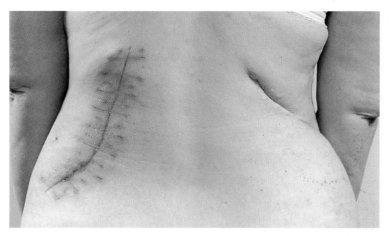

22 Female, aged 45.
(a) What is shown?
(b) What are the advantages and disadvantages of the left-sided incision?
(c) What used to be the main indication for this approach?
(d) Whose name is associated with this incision?

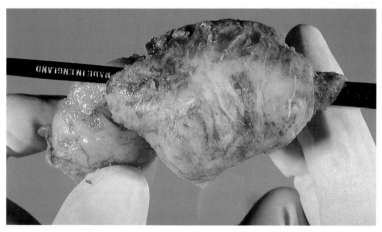

23 (a) What is this specimen?
(b) What are the common open surgical approaches to the prostate?
(c) From where is the benign adenoma thought to arise?
(d) What is Marion's sign?

24

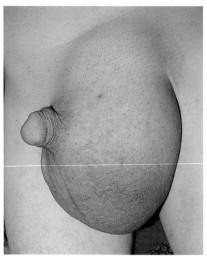

24, 25 (a) What is this lesion?
(b) How is the testis identified?
(c) What temporary manoeuvre may reduce discomfort?
(d) What procedures effect cure?
In a younger man:
(e) If a swelling is intermittent, what might this infer?
(f) Should the appearance of a swelling be regarded with suspicion?
(g) What might develop with time?

25

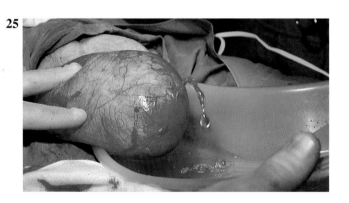

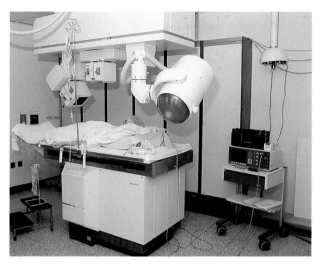

26 (a) What is this machine?
(b) How is the stone visualized?
(c) What is the advantage of this localization technique?
(d) What is the large bulbous head used for?

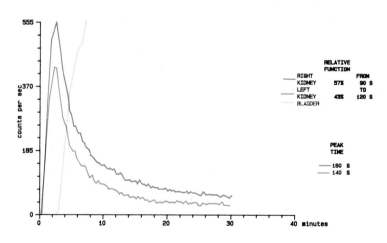

27 (a) What is this test?
(b) What is the ideal agent for assessing excretory function and what is its half life?
(c) What is the disadvantage of this agent?
(d) What phases of the curve may be recognized?

28

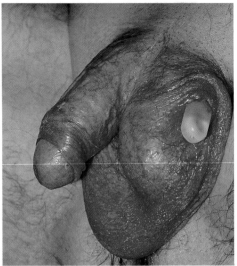

28 Male, 72, previous incontinence surgery.
(a) What is seen?
(b) What has caused this problem?
(c) What is the remedy?

29

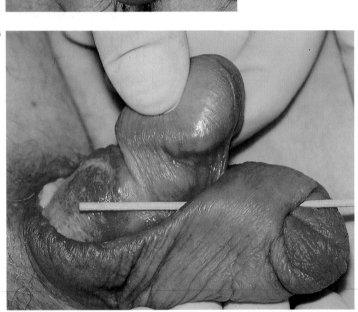

29 45-year-old male paraplegic.
(a) What has happened?

(b) Will micturition be affected?
(c) How may this be prevented?

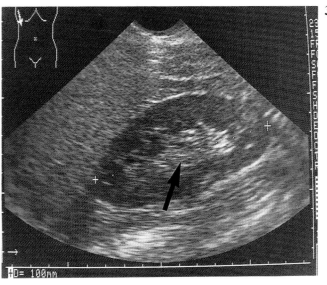

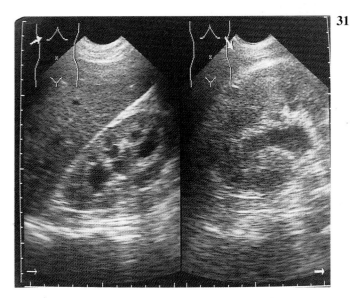

30, 31 30 is a normal ultrasound scan of a right kidney.
(a) What is the arrowed structure?
(b) What abnormal feature is present in **31**?

32

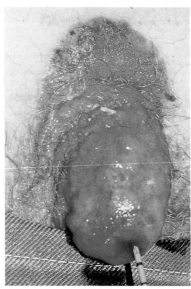

32 (a) What is this lesion?
(b) What urodynamic complication may occur?
(c) What pathological complication may occur?
(d) What further examination should be made?

33

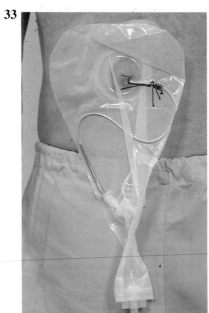

33 (a) What is this?
(b) Why is it likely to have been performed?
(c) Is general anaesthetic required?
(d) What complications may arise?

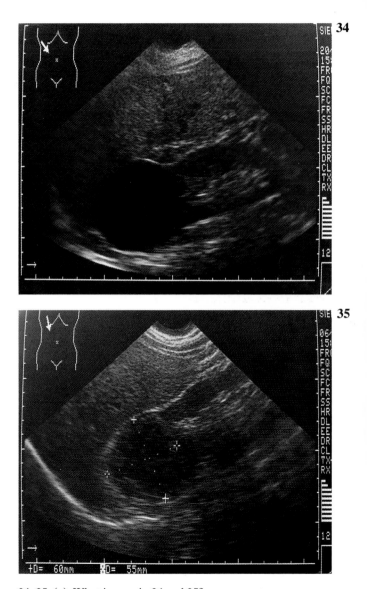

34, 35 (a) What is seen in **34** and **35**?
(b) What is the relevance of the differences between the ultrasound scans?

36

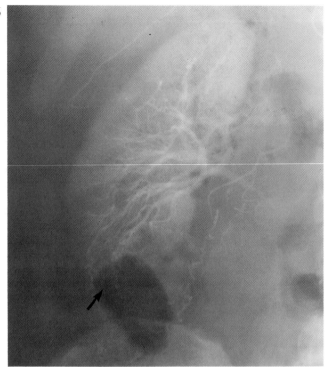

37

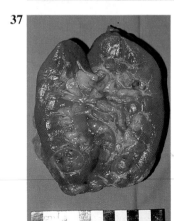

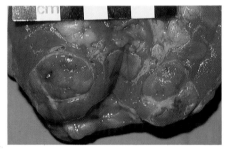

36–38 Male, aged 68, no symptoms. Lesion found on incidental ultrasound examination.
(a) What is shown?
(b) What is the likely pathology?
(c) What other pathology might be present within the kidney?
(d) What treatment is advised?

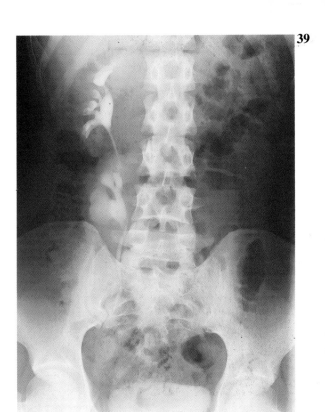

39, 40 This young patient has right iliac fossa pain.
(a) What is this condition?
(b) What is the cause of her pain?

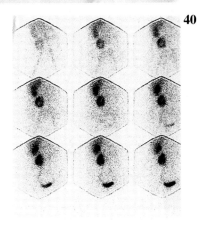

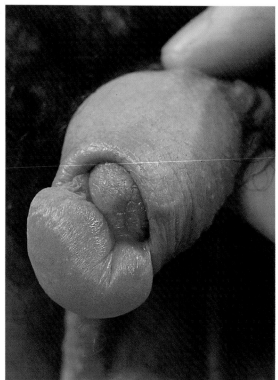

41 (a) What has recently happened?
(b) How is it likely to have been treated?
(c) What would be required if this failed?

42

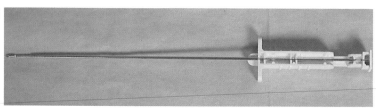

42 (a) What is this instrument?
(b) What is its common urological use?
(c) By what routes may the instrument be introduced for this purpose?
(d) What precautions may be necessary?
(e) When is this approach particularly helpful?

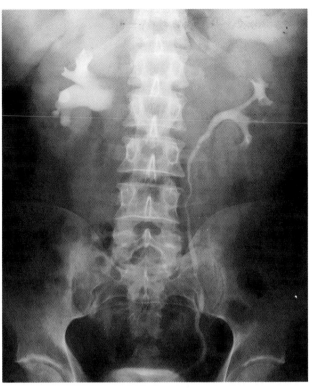

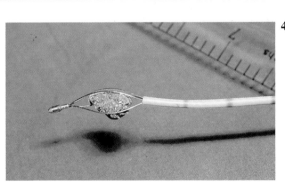

43, 44 (a) What is shown?
(b) Is urgent action required?
(c) What is this instrument called?
(d) When should it not be used?

45

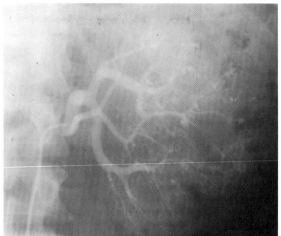

46

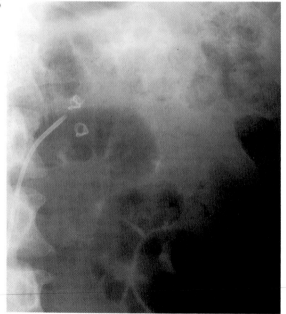

45, 46 (a) What is this examination?
(b) What does it show?
(c) What manoeuvre has been performed?
(d) What is the purpose of this?

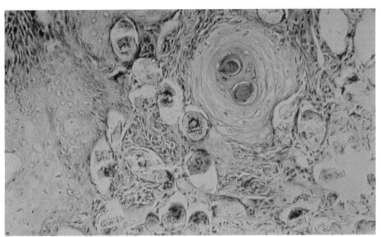

47 (a) What is this unusual bladder neoplasm?
(b) What feature is illustrated?
(c) What predisposing factors are recognized?
(d) What is the prognosis?

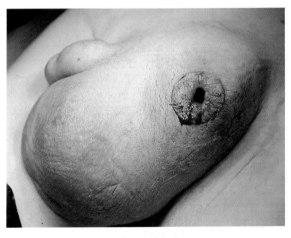

48 Male, 72, discharging faecal material.
(a) What is shown?
(b) What is the likely diagnosis?
(c) What surgical approach would be appropriate?
(d) What additional manoeuvre might be indicated?
(e) If the discharge were not faecal, what might be suspected?

49

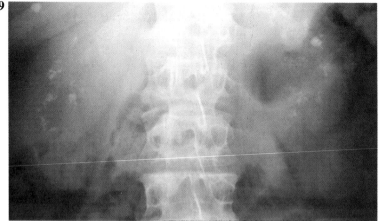

50

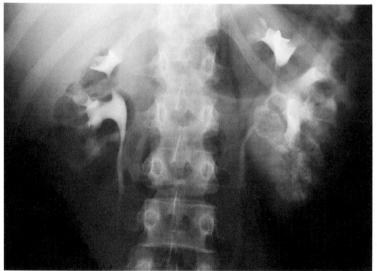

49, 50 (a) What is this condition?
(b) What is the structural abnormality?
(c) What are the radiological features?
(d) What are the complications?

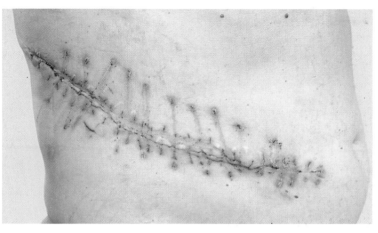

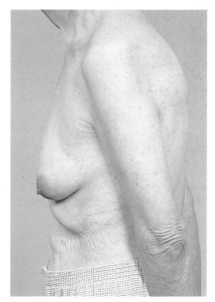

51 What problems may be associated with this loin incision:
(a) at the rear of the wound during operation?
(b) at the front of the wound during operation?
(c) in the post-operative period?
(d) in the long term?

52 Male, 78, prostate cancer.
(a) What is shown?
(b) What is the probable cause?
(c) Is this commonly seen?
(d) How may it be prevented?

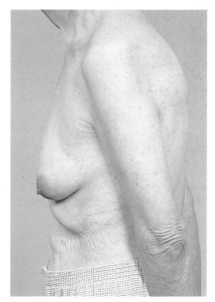

53

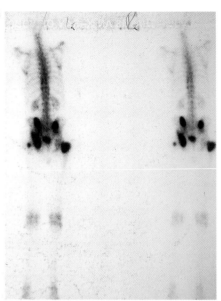

53 (a) What exactly is this test?
(b) What is the likely cause of the abnormality?
(c) What treatment is indicated?
(d) What is the approximate percentage five-year survival?

54

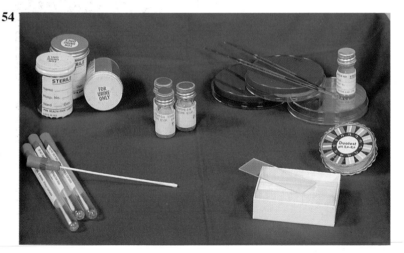

54 (a) What are these test materials used for?
(b) What does the finding of expressed prostatic fluid of pH 8 infer?
(c) What is the significance of a chlamydia serotype result positive at a dilution of 1:128?
(d) What are Vb1, Vb2 and Vb3 specimens?

IF YOU ARE TO ATTEND FOR AN I.V.P. — THAT IS AN X—RAY OF YOUR KIDNEYS AND BLADDER — DO NOT KEEP ANY RECORD ON THE DATE THAT YOU ATTEND FOR THE X—RAY EXAMINATION.

DAY	TIME / VOLUME DAY TIME (measure volumes in mls, ccs or fl. oz.)		TIME / VOLUME NIGHT TIME	
1	9.00 100 mls 10.45 50 1.30 50 3.00 50 5.00 50	7.00 100 ml 8.00 50 ml	10.00 50 mls 12.00 100 1.30 am 50 3.00 100	5.00 50 6.30 am 50
2	8.30 am 50 mls 11.00 50 12.30 100 2.30 50	4.00 50 6.00 50 8.00 50	10.00 pm 50 12.00 100 2.30 50	4.00 100 5.00 100 6.30 200
3	10 am 50 mls 1.00 20 2.30 50 5.00 100	8.00 50 mls	10.00 50 mls 1.00 am 100 2.00 100 5.00 200	7.00 100 mls 8 am 100
4	9 am 50 mls 11.00 100 1.00 100 2.00 100	4 pm 100 6.00 100 8.00 50	10.00 100 mls 12.00 100 mls 1.30 am 100 mls 3 am 100 mls	5.30 100 7.30 100
5	9.00 am - 50 mls 10.00 50 12.00 100 3.00 100	4.00 100 7.00 100	9.00 pm 100 mls 10.00 50 12.00 100 2 am 100	5.00 100 7.00 100 8.00 100
6	10 am 50 mls 12.00 100 2.00 100	4 pm 100 6.00 50 7.00 100	9.pm 100 11.00 100 1.00 100 3.00 100	6.am 100 mls
7	8 am 100 mls 9.30 50 11.30 100 1.pm 100	2.30 100 4.00 50 6.00 100 7.00 50	9.pm -100 mls 11.00 100 2.00 100 5.00 100	7 am 100 mls

♀ age 68.   Bed @ 10 pm.

55 (a) What is this chart?
(b) Why is it important?
(c) What is the normal adult physiological bladder capacity?
(d) What may be suspected if the total daily volume output is unduly high?
(e) What may be the non-urological causes of nocturia?

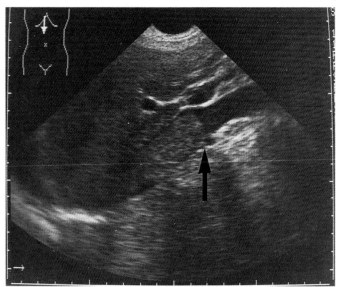

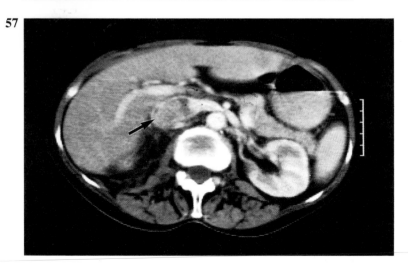

56, 57 Ultrasound and CT scan of upper abdomen.
(a) What structure is arrowed?
(b) What abnormal tissue is seen within it?
(c) What structure may be damaged during removal of this tissue?

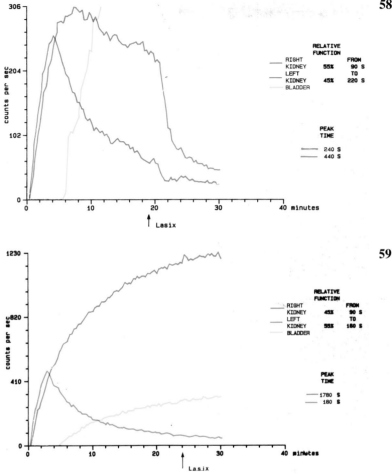

58, 59 (a) What are these investigations?
(b) What is meant by relative function?
(c) What is the purpose of administration of lasix?
(d) What is the diagnosis in each case?

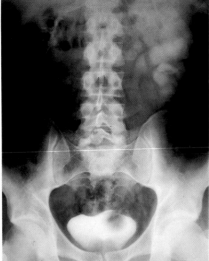

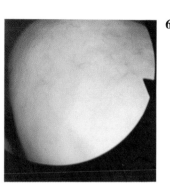
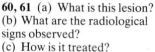

60, 61 (a) What is this lesion?
(b) What are the radiological signs observed?
(c) How is it treated?
(d) What unusual complication may occur as a result of the bladder lesion?

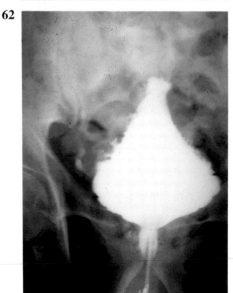

62 (a) What is seen on this micturating cysto-urethrogram?
(b) What is this commonly called?
(c) What usually gives rise to this appearance?
(d) What are the usual long-term complications to be avoided?
(e) What is the cause of the bladder wall abnormality?

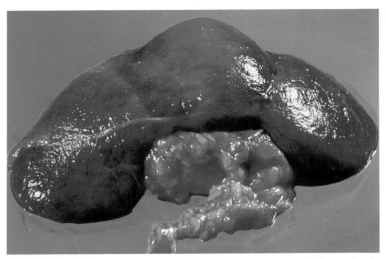

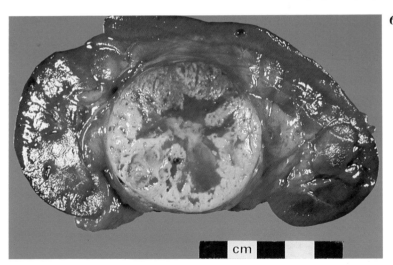

63, 64 (a) What is this lesion?
(b) What other names may describe the pathology?
(c) Why is the lesion yellow?
(d) Name two paracrine effects caused by this lesion.

65

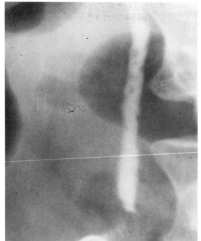

65 (a) What does this plain X-ray show?
(b) What has happened?
(c) How may this be prevented?
(d) Is treatment needed?

66

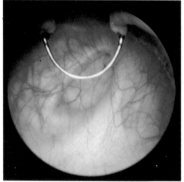

6

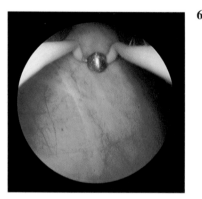

66, 67 (a) What are these endoscopic instruments?
(b) What are they used for?
(c) What fluid medium must be employed?
(d) What biochemical complication may occur after prolonged resection?

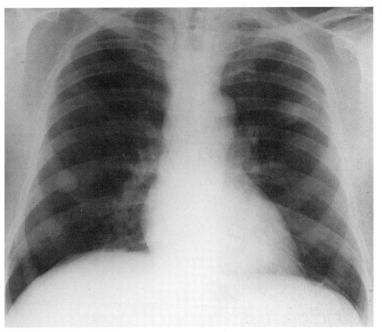

68 (a) What abnormalities are seen on this chest radiograph?
(b) What is the usual underlying lesion in adult urological patients?
(c) If a single lesion is detected, what treatment might be envisaged?

69 Male, aged 30.
(a) What is shown?
(b) What further examination should be undertaken?
(c) What tests may be required?
(d) What complications may arise as a result of this abnormality?

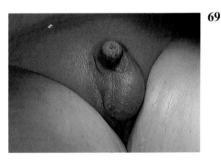

70

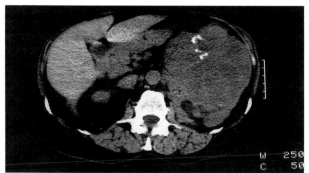

71

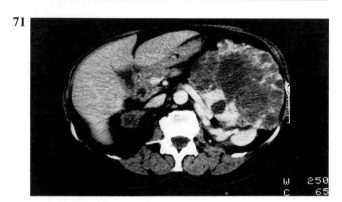

72

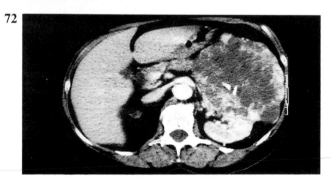

70–72 (a) What is the primary abnormality seen on the scan in **70**?
(b) What is the purpose of the supplementary scans in **71** and **72**?
(c) What major problem would occur after surgery?

73 Male, aged 24, infertile.
(a) What is this abdominal abnormality?
(b) What is the sex incidence?
(c) What is the cause of the infertility?
(d) What is an IVP likely to show?

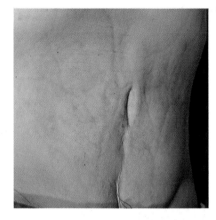

74 Traumatic haemorrhage within the perineum and scrotal wall. Will the blood pass:
(a) into the thighs?
(b) up the abdominal wall deep to Scarpa's fascia?
(c) posteriorly to surround the anus?

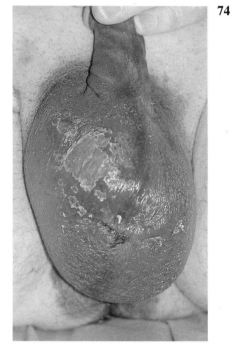

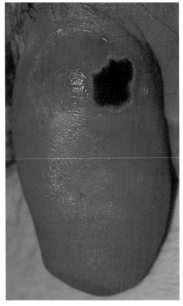

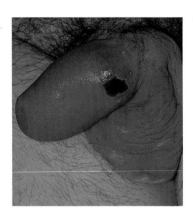

75, 76 Male, 36, diabetes-related impotence.
(a) What is illustrated?
(b) What might this condition be due to?
(c) What surgical manoeuvres are required?
(d) What further treatment should *not* be offered to this patient at a later date?

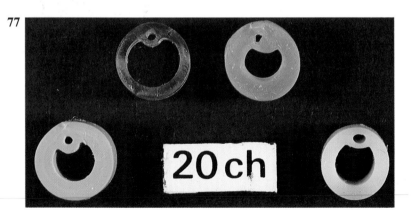

20 ch

77 (a) What are these catheters made from?
(b) What is their chief use?
(c) What is Charrière gauge?
(d) What is a coudé catheter?

78, 79 (a) What is this process?
(b) What has been the end result?
(c) What temporizing manoeuvre may sometimes be possible in this condition?

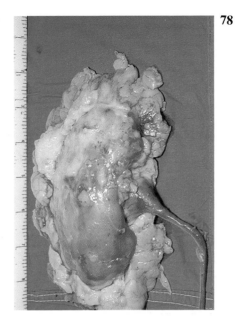

78

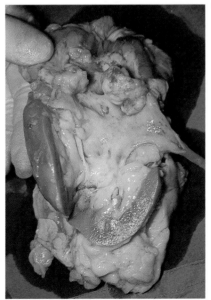

79

80

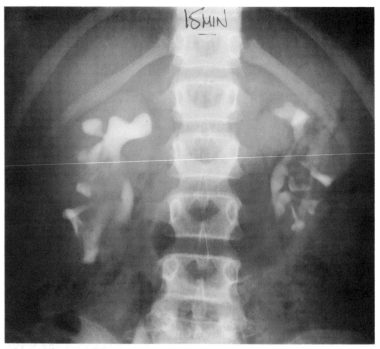

80 (a) What is this condition?
(b) What is the cardinal sign of this condition?
(c) What further radiological investigation might be considered?
(d) What is the mainstay of treatment?

81

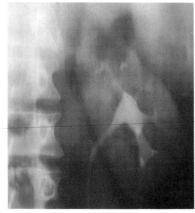

81 (a) What does this tomogram show?
(b) What is a common cause of this abnormality?
(c) What may be found in the urine?
(d) How long will confirmation of diagnosis take?

82 (a) What is seen within the bladder wall?
(b) What was its purpose?
(c) What is the active life of this treatment?
(d) What was a major drawback to the treatment?

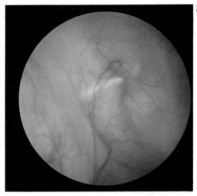

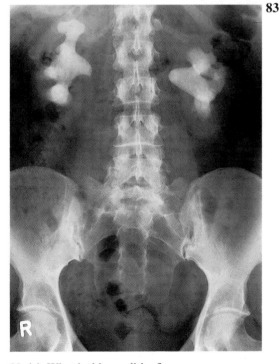

83 (a) What is this condition?
(b) What are the usual clinical presenting features?
(c) What is the modern technique of management?

84

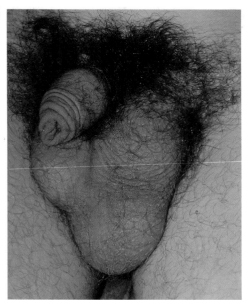

84 (a) What is this sign?
(b) What does it indicate?
(c) Is treatment necessary?

85

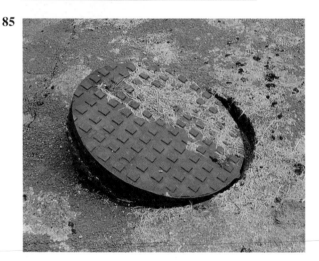

85 (a) What classical urological damage is caused by this problem?
(b) What is the nature of the damage caused?
(c) What other traumatic events may lead to the same injury?

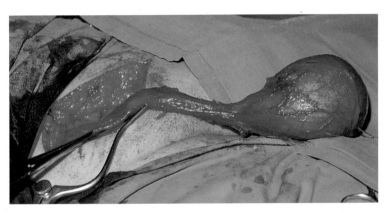

86, 87 Male aged 27.
(a) What is the likely diagnosis?
(b) What is the purpose of this particular surgical approach?
(c) What serum tests must be performed prior to surgery?
(d) Is gynaecomastia to be expected on examination?

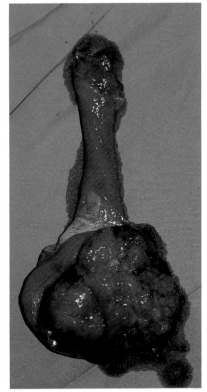

88

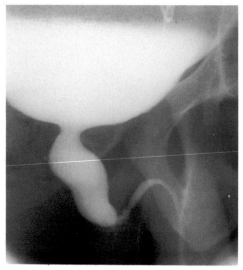

88 (a) What is this investigation?
(b) What is shown?
(c) What is the cause of the bladder neck abnormality?
(d) What treatment is required?

89

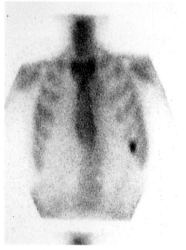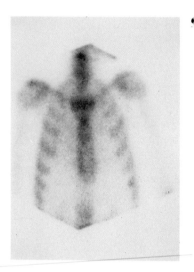

89, 90 Man aged 75, prostate cancer.
(a) What is shown in **89**?

(b) What is a possible cause?
(c) What confirmatory test is required?

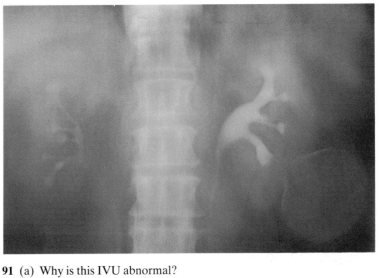

91 (a) Why is this IVU abnormal?
(b) What is the most likely cause?
(c) What are the alternative possibilities?

92 This patient has had an upper ureteric calculus.
(a) What is the tubular structure in the left upper quadrant?
(b) What subsequent treatment has occurred?
(c) How long is it reasonable to wait for recovery of renal function after treatment?

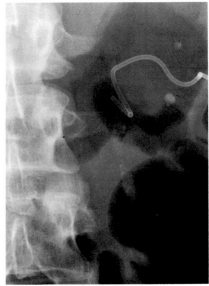

93

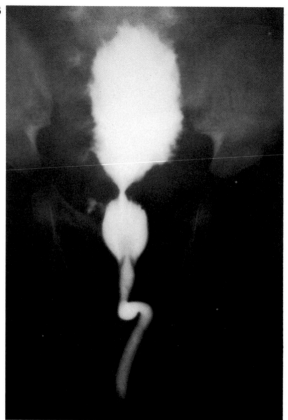

94

93, 94 (a) What is this disorder?
(b) What abnormalities are shown?
(c) What complications may
commonly occur?
(d) What is the ideal treatment?

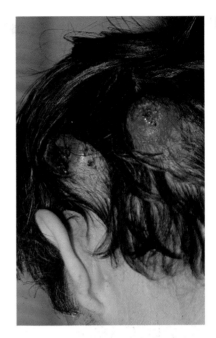

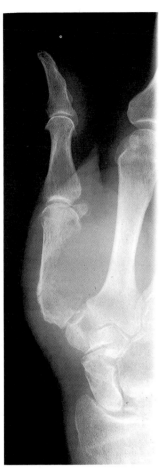

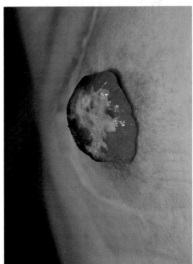

95–97 Male, aged 48, haematuria.

(a) What is the likely cause of these findings?

(b) How does this tumour frequently spread?

(c) What classical sign may occur as a result of vascular spread?

(d) What is the prognosis of this disease?

98

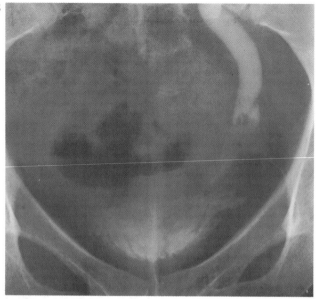

99

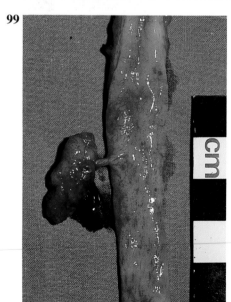

98, 99 (a) What is this lesion?
(b) What complication has occurred?
(c) What treatment can be offered?
(d) What is the prognosis?

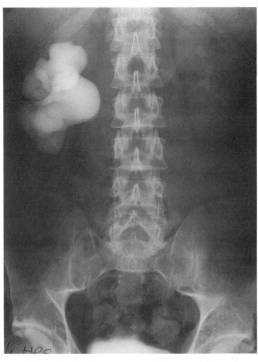

100 (a) What is the presumed diagnosis?
(b) What two other important points can be observed?
(c) What other test is required for confirmation?
(d) What is Dietl's crisis?

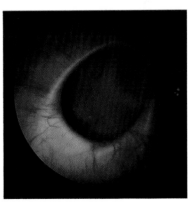

101 (a) What is seen in this endoscopic photograph?
(b) What complications may occur as a result of this finding?
(c) What investigation will demonstrate impairment of bladder function?
(d) What structure may be damaged during removal?

102

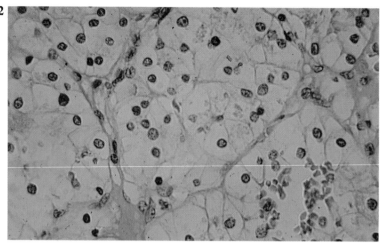

102 (a) What is this common renal tumour?
(b) What gives the cells their characteristic clear microscopic appearance?
(c) What other renal lesion may be associated?
(d) What is the relationship with the adrenal gland?

103

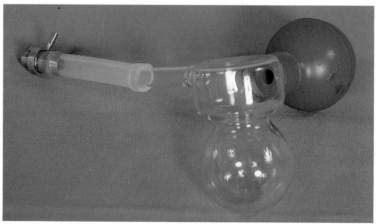

103 (a) What is this instrument?
(b) What is it used for?
(c) What complications may follow misuse?

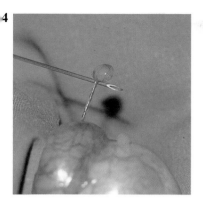

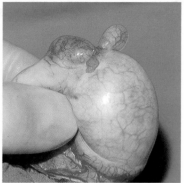

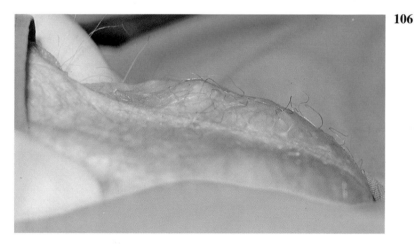

104–106 Right and left testicle from a 24-year-old.
(a) What are these structures?
(b) What may occur to them?
(c) What disorder may this mimic?
(d) From what is the testicular structure derived?

107

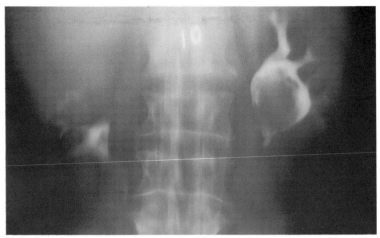

107 (a) What is observed on this tomogram?
(b) What are the treatment options?
(c) What additional investigations will be required?

108

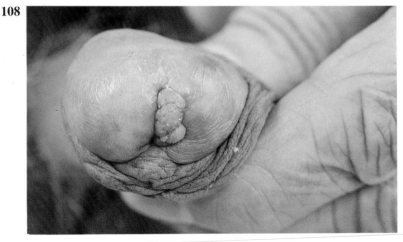

108 (a) What is this condition?
(b) How may it present?
(c) How is it treated?
(d) What complications may arise?

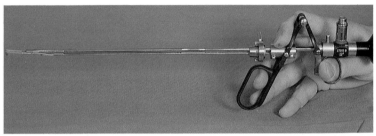

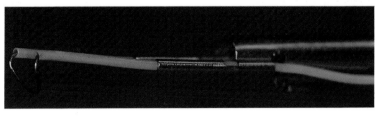

109, 110 (a) What is this surgical instrument?
(b) What are the commonly used sheath sizes?
(c) What initial procedure may be required before introduction?
(d) What common complication may follow misuse of this instrument?

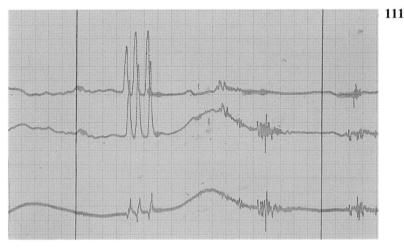

111 (a) What is this tracing?
(b) What does it show?
(c) What might the patient suffer from?
(d) What is the first line of treatment?

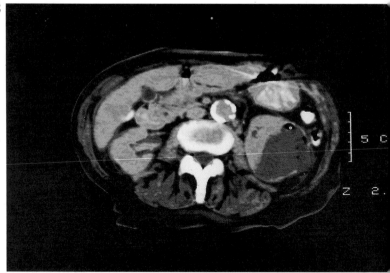

112 This elderly diabetic has a pyrexia of unknown origin and septicaemia.
(a) What abnormality is present on this CT scan?
(b) What is the diagnosis?
(c) What is the treatment?

113 (a) What is this examination?
(b) What does it show?
(c) What is the most useful further radiological investigation?

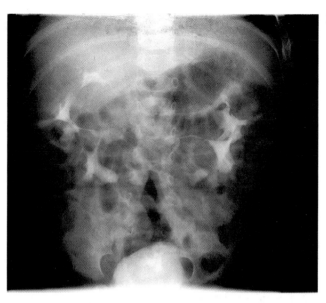

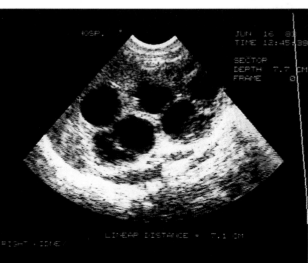

114, 115 A baby aged four months presenting with a urinary tract infection.

(a) What abnormalities are shown in the IVU and ultrasound scan?

(b) What is the diagnosis and why?

116

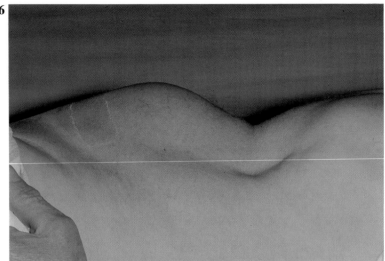

117

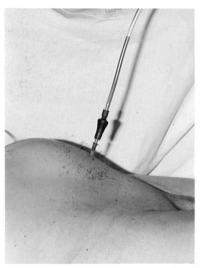

116, 117 (a) What condition do these two patients illustrate?
(b) What is the significance of the suprapubic needle and tube?
(c) What is the physiological significance of this observation?
(d) What occurs if the bladder is drained?

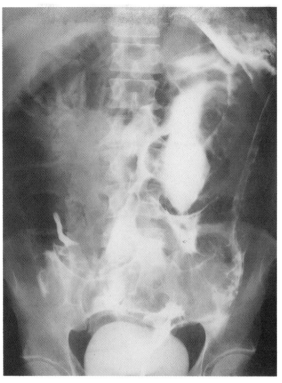

118 A driver involved in a road traffic accident.
(a) What does this X-ray show?
(b) How may this present?
(c) How has this lesion been demonstrated?
(d) How is this injury usually sustained?

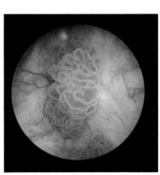

119 (a) What is this lesion?
(b) How will the patient have presented?
(c) If solitary, what is the correct
endoscopic procedure?
(d) What minimum further treatment will
be required for a low-grade tumour?

120

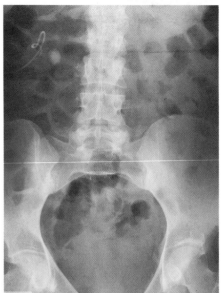

120, 121 (a) What is shown?
(b) What is the ideal treatment under these circumstances?
(c) What complications may occur during this procedure?

121

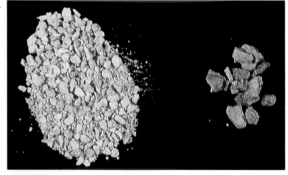

122

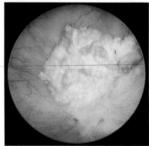

122 Male, aged 65; previous radiotherapy for invasive bladder cancer.
(a) What is seen within this bladder?
(b) What might be the cause?
(c) What further treatment is indicated?

123 Male, 72, transurethral resection of prostate.
(a) What has happened?
(b) How may this be prevented?
(c) What might the operator have noted?

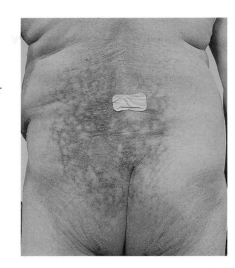

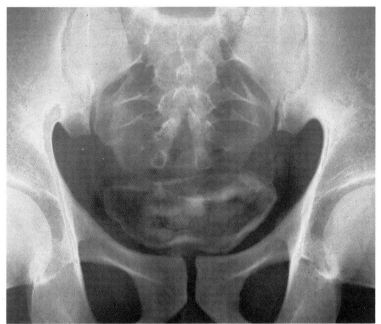

124 (a) What structure is calcified?
(b) What is the cause?
(c) What complications may eventually occur in untreated cases?

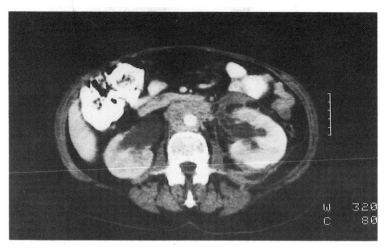

125 (a) What are the presenting clinical features of this condition, and what blood test is commonly abnormal?
(b) What abnormality is seen on this CT scan?
(c) What radiological technique may be useful in the management of such patients?
(d) What surgical procedure is performed to treat this condition?

126

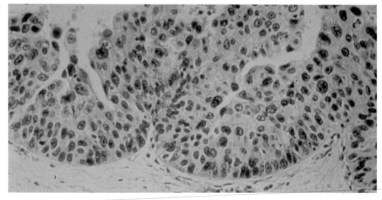

126 Bladder tumour.
(a) What is the definition of a T1 tumour?
(b) What does the prefix pT1 refer to?
(c) What is the usual initial treatment of T1 tumours?
(d) What conclusion might be drawn if hydronephrosis is present?

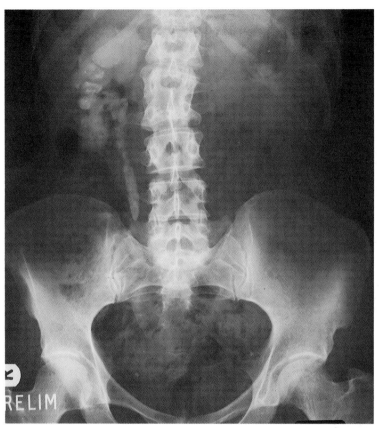

127 (a) What is the abnormality?
(b) What is the cause?
(c) What other abnormal feature is present on this radiograph?

128

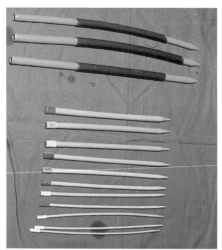

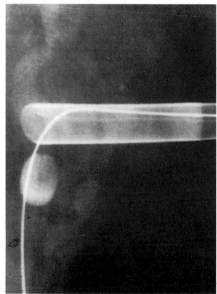

128, 129 (a) What are these instruments?
(b) What does the X-ray show?
(c) What will be the next step?
(d) Does the procedure require general anaesthetic?

129

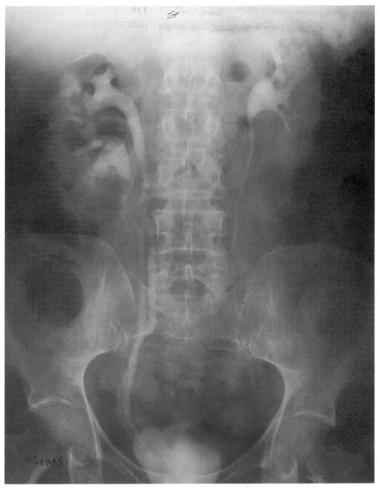

130 (a) What is the embryological origin of the ureter?
(b) What does the X-ray show?
(c) What is the relative position of the orifices within the bladder?
(d) What complication commonly occurs, related to the lower pole moiety?
(e) What may rarely cause incontinence in these patients?

131

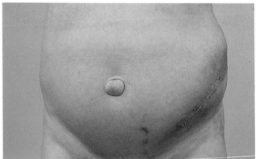

132

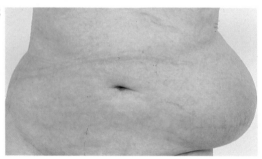

131, 132 Left renal incisions. **131**: three months post-operation. **132**: one year post-operation.
(a) What is present in these patients?
(b) What is the cause of this problem?
(c) What predisposing cause may be present?
(d) Is repair to be advised?

133

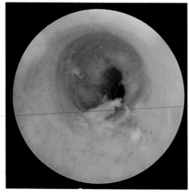

133 (a) What is shown within the urethra?
(b) What would be the characteristic appearance on uroflowmetry?
(c) After surgical treatment may the patient be discharged?
(d) What is the ideal method of follow-up?

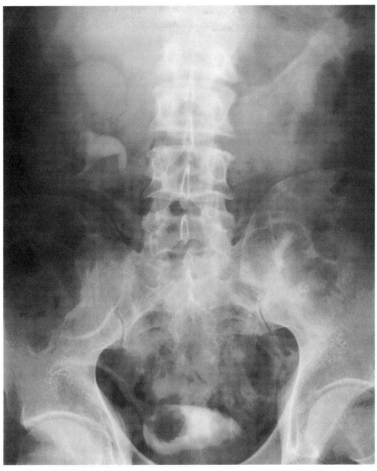

134 (a) What does this investigation demonstrate?
(b) What suggests that this may be a complex case?
(c) What further investigations are indicated?
(d) What initial treatment is required?

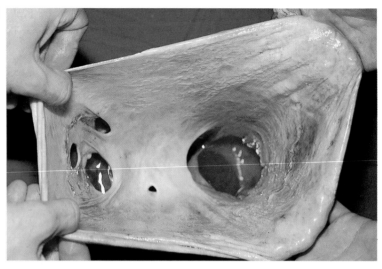

135 Male, 28 years old.
(a) What is this renal lesion, demonstrated after nephrectomy?
(b) What is the likely cause?
(c) What were the likely symptoms?

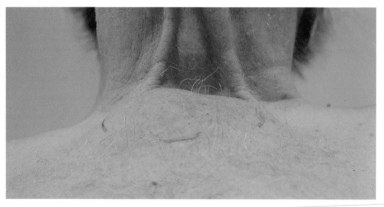

136 Male, aged 78, sudden onset of poor stream and painful sternal swelling.
(a) What is a possible diagnosis?
(b) What serum tests may be helpful?
(c) What radiological tests are required?
(d) What local treatment to the sternum may be indicated?

137 (a) What is this investigation?
(b) What does it show?
(c) What would be inferred by a history of previous urethral discharge?
(d) What is the first line of treatment?

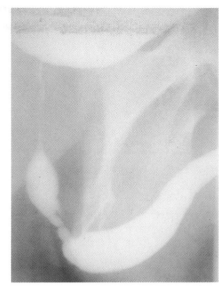

138 A section of ureter.
(a) What is shown?
(b) What predisposing factors are known?
(c) What is the connection between this disease and fishing?

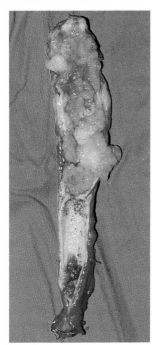

139

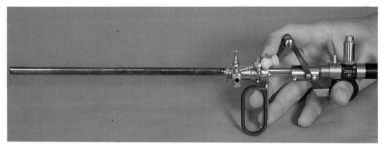

140

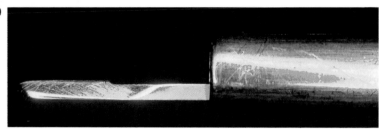

139, 140 (a) What is this instrument?
(b) What is it used for?
(c) What is the usual position for incision?
(d) What sign accompanies over-vigorous use of the instrument?

141

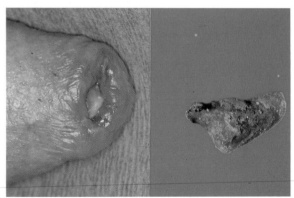

141 (a) What is this lesion?
(b) What is the predisposing cause?
(c) What additional treatment would be advisable?

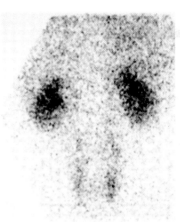
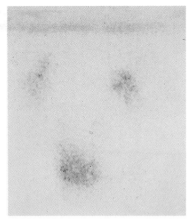

142, 143 Male, aged 36. **142**, before micturition. **143**, after micturition.
(a) What is this investigation?
(b) What is shown?
(c) What are the possible causes of this abnormality?

144 Male, grade III transitional cell carcinoma, left ureter, treated by nephro-ureterectomy eight months previously.
(a) What is this lesion?
(b) What are the likely causes?
(c) What is the prognosis of this condition?

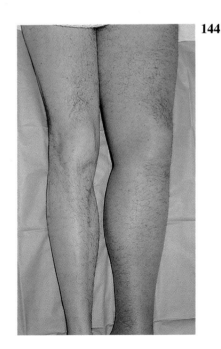

145

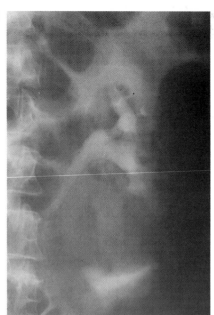

145 (a) What is the unusual feature of this IVU?
(b) What will be the likely clinical presentation?
(c) What is the cause in this case?

146

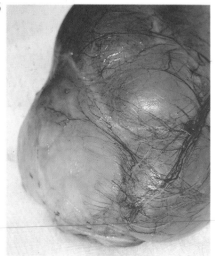

146 Scrotal contents, male aged 65.
(a) What is this disorder?
(b) How may it present?
(c) What is the diagnostic clinical sign?
(d) What is contained within?

147, 148 Male, aged 74.
(a) What is shown?
(b) What abnormal serum findings are likely?
(c) What is the likely primary?
(d) What other unrelated disorder is present within the pelvis?

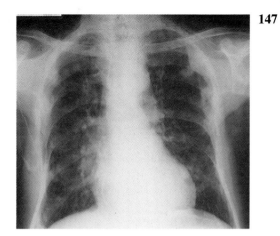

147

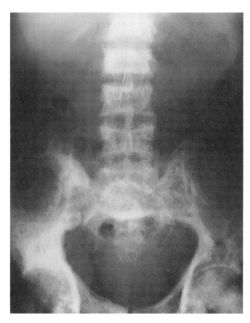

148

149 Female, aged 54, haematuria.
(a) What is the likely diagnosis?
(b) What is shown in the kidney?
(c) What factors may influence spread?
(d) What is at the lower end of the specimen?

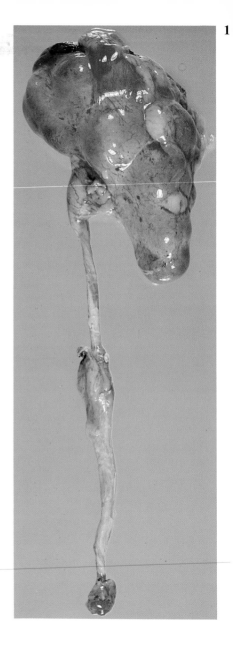

150, 151 (a) What do these X-rays show?
(b) For what purpose has this been performed?
(c) What side effects may be encountered?
(d) What may the patient notice?

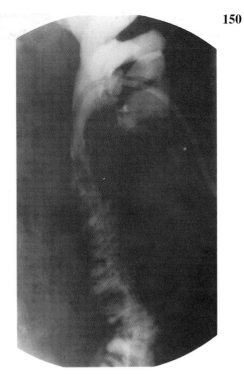

150

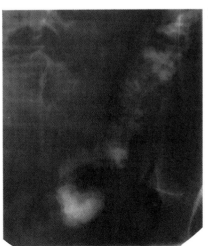

151

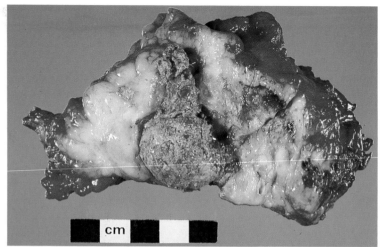

152, 153 (a) What is this disorder?
(b) What changes have occurred?
(c) What may have been the patient's symptoms?

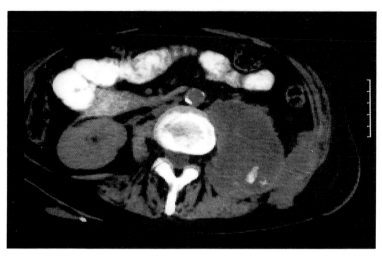

154 Female, aged 45. Previous nephrectomy for stone.
(a) What is shown?
(b) What may be the cause?
(c) What is the treatment?
(d) What is the likely outcome?

155 Male, aged 34 years.
(a) What is shown on this IVP?
(b) What is the likely diagnosis?
(c) What simple test will demonstrate the abnormality?
(d) What renal abnormality may occasionally occur?

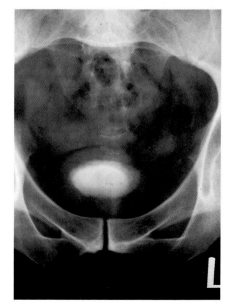

156

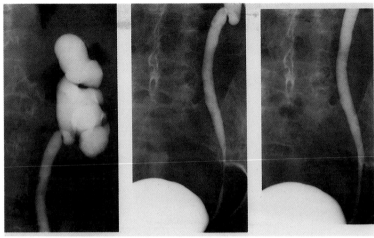

156 (a) What is this test?
(b) What has it shown?
(c) Is surgical treatment usually required in the adult?
(d) What are the common complications?

157

157 (a) What systemic alkylator treatment is likely to have been given to this patient?
(b) What is the chief urological symptom?
(c) What other complications may occur?

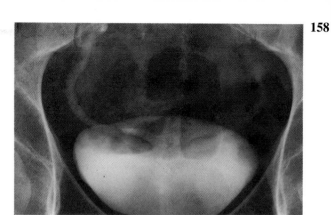

158 (a) What are the abnormalities?
(b) Why does this appearance occur?
(c) What symptoms might be present?
(d) What percentage are bilateral?

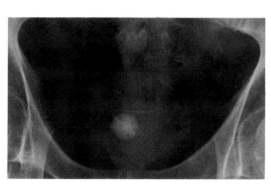

159, 160 (a) What is shown on this plain X-ray?
(b) What is the classical symptom produced by the lesion?
(c) What surgical procedure will be required?

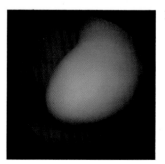

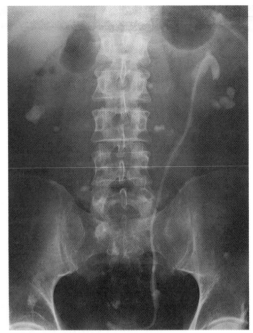

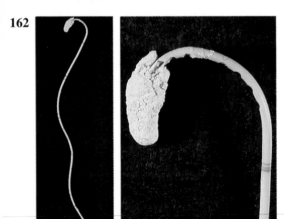

161, 162 (a) What has occurred in this 'stone forming' patient?
(b) How can this situation best be resolved?
(c) What is the usual method of stent removal?

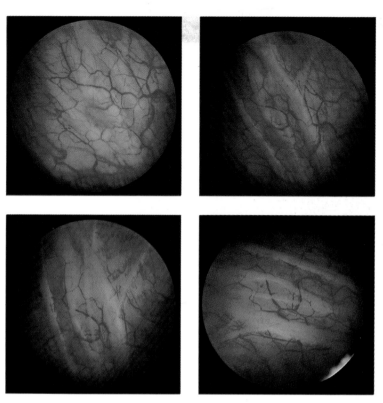

163 Bladder wall photographed empty (top left); with 150 ml (top right); with 250 ml (bottom left); and with 400 ml contained within.
(a) What is observed?
(b) What may be the composition of the trabecular bars?
(c) What is the effect of severe obstruction?

164

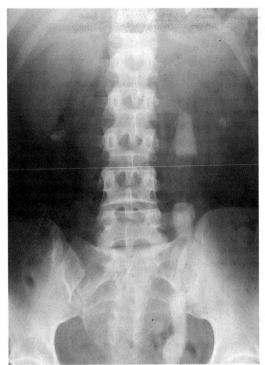

164 (a) What does this plain film show?
(b) What is the probable underlying disorder?
(c) What further tests will be required to clarify
the diagnosis?
(d) If renography is considered, what
precautions will be required during
analysis?

165

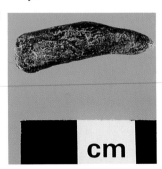

165 Recovered from the bladder two
years after prostatectomy.
(a) What is this likely to be?
(b) How would it present?
(c) Which patients are prone to this
problem?

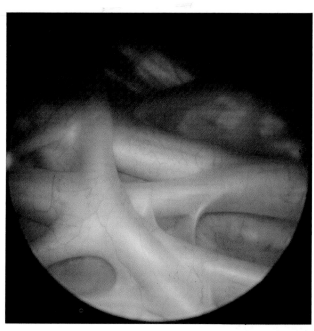

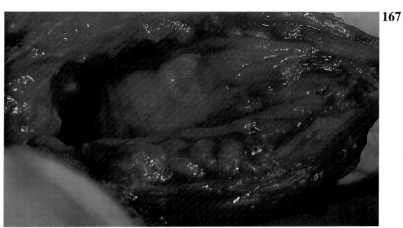

166, 167 (a) What does this endoscopic picture show?
(b) A grossly thickened bladder wall (seen at open operation) is typical of what disorders?
(c) What may be the effect on upper tracts?

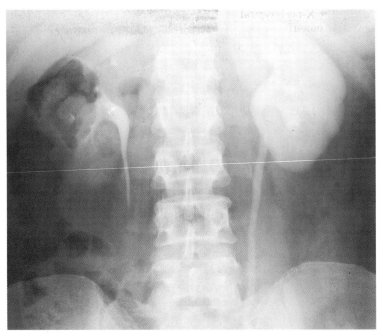

168 (a) What does this film show?
(b) What does this mean?
(c) What are the likely causes?

169

169 (a) What is this neoplastic lesion seen within the urethra?
(b) How are such lesions best observed?
(c) What implication does this finding carry for the remainder of the urinary tract?
(d) How might this finding affect the available surgical options?

170 (a) The X-ray is typical of what condition?
(b) What are the other cardinal signs of this condition?
(c) What treatment is required?
(d) What is the outcome if the patient remains untreated?

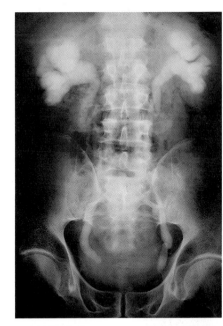

171 (a) What does this IVP show?
(b) What biochemical abnormality may arise and under what circumstances?
(c) For what disease is this procedure most commonly performed?
(d) What minor procedure is carried out at the same time as the major surgery to anticipate possible future complications?

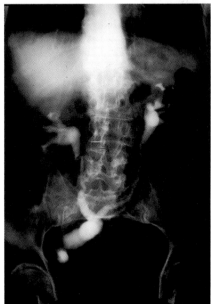

172

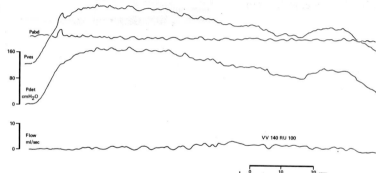

173

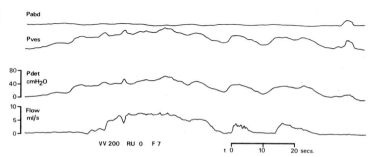

172, 173 (a) What are these tests?
(b) Why is an abdominal (rectal) pressure line required?
(c) What does each test illustrate?

174, 175 Male, resident in tropics.
(a) What is the likely diagnosis?
(b) What is the causative organism?
(c) What may the blood picture show?
(d) What is the ideal local treatment?
(e) What systemic agent is available for treatment?

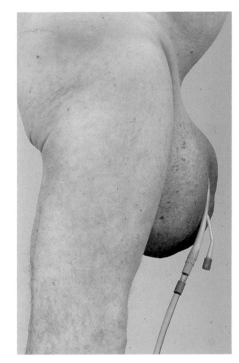

174

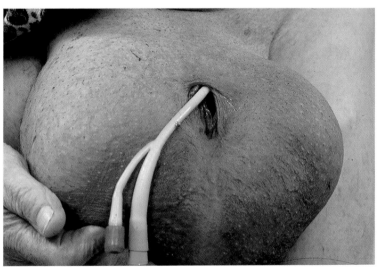

175

176

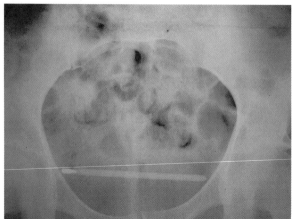

177

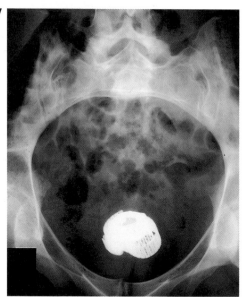

178

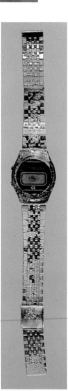

176–178 (a) What is shown within the bladder?
(b) How did the patients present?
(c) Where might such patients have originated?
(d) What lesson is illustrated by these findings?

179, 180 (a) What is the diagnosis?
(b) When does this classically occur?
(c) What warning signs may have been present?
(d) What operative manoeuvre must be performed?

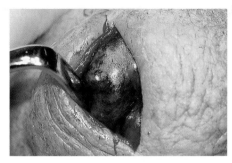

179

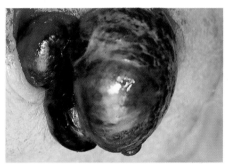

180

181 Female, aged 40, no neurological signs.
(a) What is this investigation?
(b) What is the possible cause?
(c) What is the possible consequence?
(d) What is the ideal treatment?

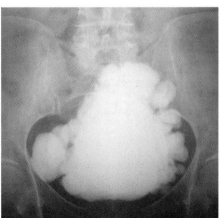

181

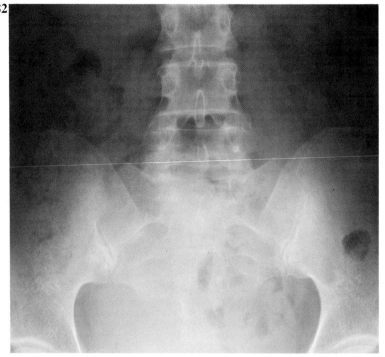

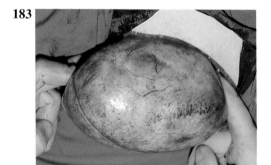

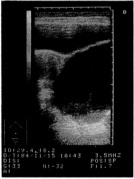

182–184 Female, aged 48. Findings at laparotomy.
(a) What is this lesion?
(b) What is a likely mode of presentation?
(c) What vital structure is at risk during removal?
(d) What complication must be avoided during removal?

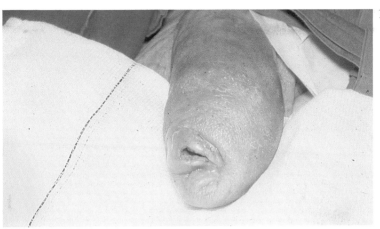

185, 186 (a) What is this lesion?
(b) How may it have presented?
(c) What precaution should be taken before assessing spread?
(d) What is the treatment?
(e) What local complication may arise after surgery?

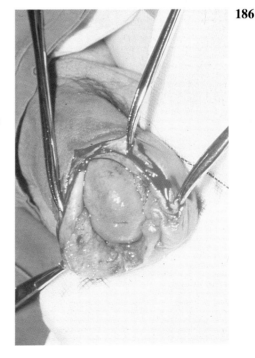

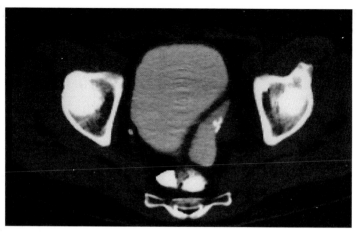

187 (a) What does this CT scan illustrate?
(b) What is seen within the lesion?
(c) What might this indicate?
(d) What is the prognosis?

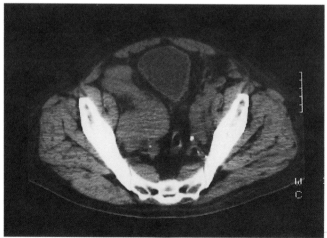

188 Male, aged 71, firm prostate.
(a) What is shown?
(b) How may this often present?
(c) What will the bone scan show?
(d) Is treatment effective?

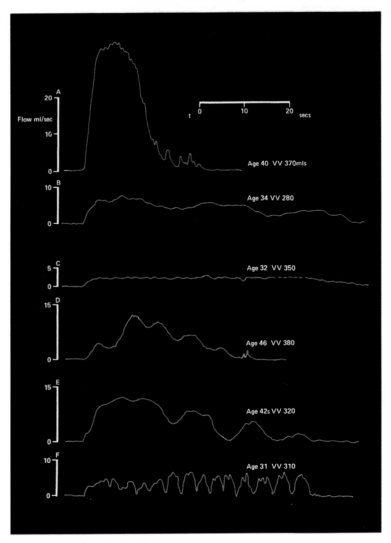

189 Various uroflow rates. What do A–F show?

190

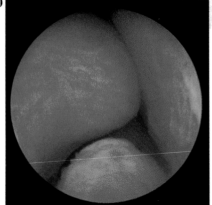

190 Male, aged 74. Endoscopic view from the level of external sphincters.
(a) What is seen?
(b) Is prostatic size related to the patient's symptoms?
(c) What is the importance of the landmarks identified?
(d) What sexual dysfunction should be mentioned to the patient before prostatectomy?

191

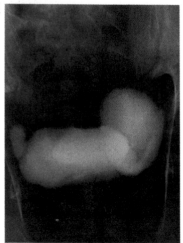

1

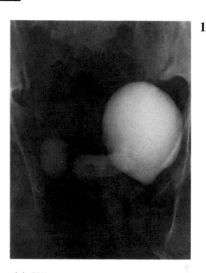

191, 192 (a) What is this investigation?
(b) What is shown?

(c) What symptom would the patient suffer?
(d) What treatment is advised?

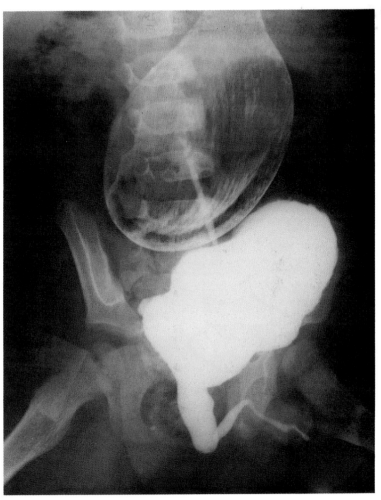

193 (a) What is this test?
(b) What is the purpose of the manoeuvre?
(c) What is the purpose of the spoon?
(d) What is the main drawback of the test?

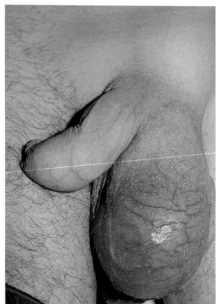

194

194, 195 Male, age 64,
symptoms of three months'
duration.
(a) What is shown?
(b) What is the likely
diagnosis?
(c) What other radiological
investigations are required?
(d) What is the prognosis?

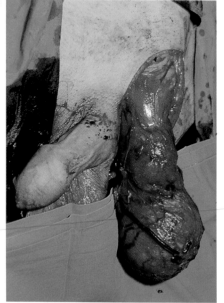

195

ANSWERS

1, 2 (a) Horseshoe kidney. The lower poles of the kidneys are displaced towards the mid-line and are joined by a bridge of functioning renal tissue or a fibrous band, crossing in front of the aorta, inferior vena cava and spine.
(b) Stasis of contrast within the pelvicalyceal systems. This is a consequence of the associated malrotation of the kidney, the pelvis lying anteriorly rather than medially. The upper ureters are required to pass over the isthmus before taking up a normal path.
(c) Infection and stone formation as a complication of the stasis.
(d) A renal cell carcinoma at its superolateral aspect.

3, 4 (a) Congenital pelviureteric junction (PUJ) obstruction.
(b) No transmission of urine across the PUJ despite overdistended pelvis (transilluminated for clarity).
(c) Loin pain especially after drinking; haematuria; infection; stone formation.
(d) Pyeloplasty (obviously nephrectomy was performed in this case, for poor function) of which the common operations are the Anderson–Hynes (dismembered) pyeloplasty and the Culp (flap) pyeloplasty.

5 (a) Hypernephroma.
(b) Haematuria, upper quadrant pain and mass.
(c) Pyrexia of unknown origin, weight loss, polycythaemia or anaemia.
(d) Ultrasound scanning to differentiate between solid and cystic mass.

6 (a) Squamous cell carcinoma scrotum.
(b) Local exposure to soot, oil or petroleum products.
(c) Radical local excision.
(d) Perineal urethrostomy.

7 (a) *Herpes Zoster.*
(b) It can occur with a widespread spinal malignant process.
(c) Before vesicles erupt, pain may lead to a false diagnosis of advancing skeletal disease.
(d) Is there recent family history of chicken pox?

8 (a) Wilms' tumour (nephroblastoma).
(b) Up to 5 years.
(c) Increased abdominal girth or abdominal mass (pain and bleeding are unusual).
(d) Lung; bone, liver and lymph nodes may also be involved.

9, 10 (a) Adenocarcinoma of the bladder.
(b) Rare — 1% of bladder tumours.
(c) Vault (urachus); hence of glandular origin.
(d) Radical excisional surgery (illustrated) to include the umbilicus.

11, 12 (a) Large kidneys with distortion of the pelvicalyceal system, due to adult type of polycystic disease.
(b) Ultrasound scanning of kidneys, liver and pancreas, all of which may contain cysts.
(c) Autosomal dominant, in contradistinction to infantile polycystic disease, which is autosomal recessive.
(d) Loin pain, abdominal mass, hypertension, renal failure or haematuria.

13 (a) Oxalate calculus.
(b) Urinary infection, particularly with urea-splitting organisms, such as proteus.
(c) Common in children in India and the Middle East; common in male elderly adults in the Western world (outflow tract obstruction).
(d) Diverticulum of the bladder (stasis).

14 (a) Large 'floppy' low pressure chronic retention.
(b) Poor stream; straining; recurrent urinary infection.
(c) Treatment (transurethral resection (TUR) and/or bladder reduction operations) rarely restores normal function to the overstretched detrusor muscle.
(d) Renal function is usually *not* affected as the low intrinsic bladder pressure does not threaten the upper tracts.

15, 16 (a) Left hydronephrosis. Right filling defect upper pole; probably transitional cell carcinoma. Two lesions (transitional cell carcinoma (TCC)) are seen in the specimen — the smaller is indicated by the probe.
(b) Haematuria.
(c) Nephro-ureterectomy (R) after the cause of the left (incidental in this case) hydronephrosis has been diagnosed.
(d) Review cystoscopies.

17, 18 (a) Balanitis xerotica obliterans.
(b) Painful phimosis or urethral stenosis with consequent urethral obstruction.
(c) Circumcision may alleviate discomfort related to the foreskin, but pathology involving the urethra (illustrated) is common and requires regular dilatation.

19 (a) Seminoma of testis.

(b) Lymphatic to para-aortic glands.

(c) Typically sheets of round cells with clear cytoplasm and large nuclei.

(d) Radiotherapy — highly radiosensitive tumour.

20, 21 (a) Pelvic kidney, this being single in **21**. The foetal kidney develops within the pelvis and ascends to its normal position in the upper abdomen.

(b) Lower abdominal mass or pyelonephritis.

(c) From the iliac arteries or lower abdominal aorta.

22 (a) Right — conventional loin incision; Left — lumbotomy approach (slightly hook-ended inferiorly).

(b) Less pain, more restricted access, difficult in fat patients.

(c) Before percutaneous surgery and lithotripsy this limited approach was often used to remove pelvic calculi. It is not suitable for any major operation on the kidney.

(d) Gil-Vernet, whose name is also given to the special retractors required for the operation.

23 (a) Open prostatectomy specimen showing lateral lobes and a smaller middle lobe; pencil indicates course of the urethra.

(b) Transvesical or retropubic (Millin) prostatectomy.

(c) From para-urethral glands.

(d) A markedly enlarged middle lobe prevents the ureteric orifices from being viewed at cystoscopy.

24, 25 (a) Hydrocele — straw coloured fluid being drained prior to corrective surgery.

(b) By transillumination; the testis cannot be palpated (contrast epididymal cyst).

(c) Needle aspiration (avoiding blood vessels by transillumination) and possibly by instilling tetracycline into the sac.

(d) Sac may be excised (Jaboulay) or incised and plicated (Lord).

(e) Patent processus vaginalis (i.e. persistent congenital hydrocele).

(f) Yes — there may be an underlying disease such as testicular tumour.

(g) Hernia down patent processus.

26 (a) Lithotriptor — extra corporeal shock wave (Siemens).

(b) By X-ray control (X-ray head above table).

(c) X-ray visualization allows ureteric stones to be treated as well as renal calculi (ureteric stones are difficult to localize with ultrasound).

(d) Ultrasonic localization of gall bladder calculi.

27 (a) Isotope renogram.

(b) ^{123}ortho-iodohippurate (OIH); 13 hours.

(c) Expensive; it has to be produced in a cyclotron and thus availability is a problem.

(d) Three phases: First, vascular; second, renal handling of OIH; third, excretory — the third phase should be concave, as illustrated.

28 (a) A silicone pump of artificial sphincter is seen protruding through the left neck of the scrotum.

(b) Infection likely, although sterile pressure necrosis can cause mechanical parts to ulcerate to the skin surface.

(c) Removal of the entire apparatus.

29 (a) Pressure necrosis of penile skin has allowed the glans to dislocate through the defect. The marker shows the correct position.

(b) No — urethral elements are not affected.

(c) Regular attention to pressure areas below the sensory level.

30, 31 (a) The normal central echo complex, consisting of the pelvicalyceal system, vascular structures and sinus fat.

(b) This kidney is hydronephrotic, the central echo complex being separated by excess fluid within the collecting system.

32 (a) Paget's disease of the penis (erythroplasia of Queyrat).

(b) Urethral stenosis: stricture.

(c) Carcinoma of the penis.

(d) Regional (inguinal) lymph nodes must be examined.

33 (a) Percutaneous nephrostomy, left kidney.

(b) Hydronephrosis or pyonephrosis with distal obstruction.

(c) No — it can be placed under local anaesthetic.

(d) Haemorrhage during passage — not usually serious. Infection of tract and urine — usually with skin organisms, such as *S. aureus*.

34, 35 (a) **34** shows a simple renal cyst; **35** shows a solid lesion.
(b) Simple cysts are common and are rarely of clinical significance. The solid lesion is a renal tumour requiring further investigation and treatment.

36–38 (a) Abnormal circulation pattern, lower pole.
(b) Hypernephroma — small encapsulated lesion seen within the lower pole.
(c) Other adenomata may be found in association with the tumour.
(d) Nephrectomy.

39, 40 (a) Crossed ectopic kidney. Congenitally both kidneys are on the same side of the body, although the ureter of the lower kidney will cross the mid-line in order to enter the bladder trigone on the correct side.
(b) Obstruction of the urine outflow from the lower kidney, due to an anomalous blood vessel, which commonly occurs in positional abnormalities of the kidneys.

41 (a) Recent reduction of paraphimosis — oedema of prepuce.
(b) Gentle pressure with a cold wet swab over 10–15 minutes.
(c) Operative reduction under anaesthesia with elective circumcision (difficult to achieve a good result with gross oedema present).

42 (a) Trucut biopsy needle.
(b) Biopsy of prostate gland.
(c) Transperineal; transrectal.
(d) Antibiotics will be required to cover use via the transrectal route (septicaemia).
(e) In early prostate cancer: this disease starts in the periphery of the gland and is amenable to needle biopsy diagnosis before histology can be obtained by the transurethral route.

43, 44 (a) Hydronephrosis, presumed due to the lower ureteric stone.
(b) Not on this evidence — calyces cupped and further films may show passage of contrast down the ureter.
(c) Dormia basket.
(d) When used blind (without a ureteroscope) the basket should not be used more than 5 cm up the ureter.

45, 46 (a) Left selective renal arteriogram.

(b) Tumour circulation — presumed hypernephroma.

(c) Vascular occlusion by coil embolization (coils visible).

(d) To reduce vascular supply to the tumour; induce immunological reaction to the tumour (effect not proven).

47 (a) Squamous cell carcinoma of the bladder.

(b) Keratin pearl formation.

(c) Chronic inflammatory disorders, e.g. bladder stone, schistosomiasis.

(d) Usually poor: pearl formation is, however, a sign of good differentiation in squamous cell tumours.

48 (a) Fistula in the left hemi-scrotum.

(b) Obstructed and/or strangulated bowel in the hernia sac.

(c) Abdominal approach will isolate the strangulated loop and prevent contamination prior to removal of the necrotic scrotal contents.

(d) Left orchidectomy to allow adequate repair of the defect in the abdominal wall.

(e) Tuberculosis — chronic discharging epididymitis.

49, 50 (a) Medullary sponge kidney; this is commonly bilateral, but may be unilateral.

(b) Congenital ectasia of the tubules in the medullary pyramids.

(c) Nephrocalcinosis in the region of the pyramids, contrast filling of the ectatic tubules and large kidneys.

(d) Infection and the passage of calculi.

51 (a) Pleural space may be entered.

(b) Peritoneum and ascending colon may interfere with access.

(c) Pain may prevent adequate thoracic excursion, leading to chest infection.

(d) Such wounds may be uncomfortable for many weeks — a manual worker may be off work for up to three months.

52 (a) Gynaecomastia.

(b) Oestrogen treatment for metastatic disease.

(c) No, as oestrogens are contraindicated due to side effects from fluid retention.

(d) Radiotherapy to breasts can prevent symptoms if oestrogen must be given.

53 (a) Radioisotope bone scan.
(b) Prostate cancer.
(c) Hormonal manipulation — orchidectomy and/or LHRH agonists or anti-androgen therapy.
(d) 10–14%.

54 (a) Testing for prostatic infection — routine urine culture pots, Stuart's transport media, pH papers, slides for direct microscopy and culture media for chlamydia trachomatis.
(b) Present or past infection in prostate fluid — inflammatory exudate alters pH from the normal range of 6.5–7.1.
(c) Present *or past* exposure to *C. Trachomatis* — this finding does *not* necessarily infer active infection at present.
(d) Voided bladder specimens. Vb1, initial stream (urethral washout); Vb2, mid-stream urine (bladder); Vb3, post-prostatic massage urine (organisms expressed from prostatic ducts).

55 (a) Frequency volume chart of urine excreted over a seven-day period.
(b) It gives essential objective information on a patient's micturition habit.
(c) 400–550 ml.
(d) Polyuria — excessive drinking, diabetes mellitus or insipidus, etc.
(e) Heart failure; renal failure; evening diuretic medication.

56, 57 (a) Inferior vena cava.
(b) Secondary spread via the renal vein from a hypernephroma — may be blood clot or tumour.
(c) The opposite renal vein.

58, 59 (a) Diuretic renograms.
(b) The function of each kidney relative to the other — total glomerular filtration rate (GFR) is required to assess the quantitative function overall.
(c) To determine the difference between the large non-obstructed 'baggy' system and the truly obstructed renal pelvis.
(d) **58** 'Baggy'. **59** Completely obstructed (no drainage after lasix).

60, 61 (a) Large ureterocele.
(b) Space-occupying lesion within the bladder, hydronephrosis.
(c) Resection of the ureterocele wall.
(d) Bladder neck obstruction due to ureterocele prolapse.

62 (a) Thick walled, conical, heavily trabecular bladder.
(b) Fir-tree bladder.
(c) Neurological (reflex) bladder disorder.
(d) Hydronephrosis; renal failure.
(e) Intermittent detrusor contraction against closed urethral sphincter (dyssynergia).

63, 64 (a) Hypernephroma.
(b) Von Grawitz tumour, adenocarcinoma, clear cell carcinoma.
(c) Lipid within the cytoplasm.
(d) Erythropoietin (red cell mass raised) and parathyroid hormone (hypercalcaemia) production.

65 (a) Steinstrasse.
(b) Lithotripsy to stone in the kidney or upper ureter — good result but fragments have accumulated in the ureter.
(c) Diuresis during extra-corporeal shock wave lithotrypsy (ESWL); stent *in situ*.
(d) Yes — steinstrasses will coalesce if not broken up (i.e., within two weeks).

66, 67 (a) Resectoscope cutting loop and ball diathermy electrode.
(b) Transurethral resection of bladder lesions and/or prostate and subsequent electrocoagulation of bleeding vessels.
(c) Fluid must be near-isotonic (prevent haemolysis if absorbed) and not conduct electric current (dissipates cutting or coagulation effect).
(d) TUR 'syndrome' — influx of irrigation fluid through open vessels leading to dilutional hyponatraemia.

68 (a) 'Cannon ball' pulmonary metastases.
(b) Classically, hypernephroma; occasionally, seminoma.
(c) Lobectomy — patients may have long-term survival after removal of single metastases from hypernephroma.

69 (a) Cryptorchidism, right side. Absent hemi-scrotum confirms that the testis has never descended.
(b) Careful examination of the groin for signs of arrested descent — it cannot be brought into the scrotum.
(c) CT scan or laparoscopy may identify testis or gonadal vessels on the posterior abdominal wall.
(d) Torsion (occasional), malignant change (rare, but increased risk of change).

70–72 (a) Left renal tumour with calcification.
(b) To observe enhancement of the tumour, demonstrate the normality of the left renal vein and inferior vena cava and to locate sites of spread to local lymph nodes and/or psoas muscles.
(c) Renal failure; the right kidney is small, atrophic and non-functioning.

73 (a) Prune belly syndrome.
(b) Almost exclusively male.
(c) Bilateral cryptorchidism is the rule.
(d) Bilateral hydronephrosis.

74 (a) No — Scarpa's fascia prevents downwards spread — attached at top of thigh.
(b) Yes.
(c) No — attachment of the perineal fascia to the posterior aspect of the urologenital diaphragm prevents spread posteriorly.

75, 76 (a) Acute inflammation and abscess formation in the left corpus cavernosum.
(b) Self injection with papaverine for treatment of impotence.
(c) Incision; drainage; urethroscopy to ensure that the urethra is not compromised.
(d) Insertion of penile prosthesis — this will almost certainly fail due to infection and/or abscess formation.

77 (a) (From left) silicone coated latex (Silastic^{TM}); plastic; latex rubber; pure silicone.
(b) Silicone catheters, long-term urinary drainage; plastic catheter (large lumen), post-operative drainage; latex catheter, short-term drainage of debris-free urine (small lumen).
(c) Circumference in millimetres (Joseph Charrière).
(d) Catheter with a terminal bend (coudé = elbow) to help pass over the bladder neck.

78, 79 (a) Obstruction (upper pole); infection; necrosis.
(b) Necrotic pyonephrosis.
(c) Percutaneous drainage of infected pyonephrosis.

80 (a) Pyelonephritis.
(b) Loss of cortical thickness opposite the calyx.
(c) Micturating cystogram — for reflux.
(d) Accurate bacteriological localization and antibiotic therapy.

81 (a) Stenosis of the neck of the upper pole calyx.
(b) Tuberculosis.
(c) Sterile pyuria.
(d) Confirmatory cultures require six weeks' incubation.

82 (a) Radioactive gold grain (^{198}Au).
(b) Treatment of bladder tumour (no longer used).
(c) Half life of ^{198}Au is 60 h.
(d) Difficult to localize grains within the tumour base.

83 (a) Bilateral staghorn calculi.
(b) Loin pain, recurrent infections, haematuria or renal impairment.
(c) Percutaneous debulking of the calculi, followed by lithotripsy of any remaining fragments.

84 (a) 'Pawnbroker' sign — discrete lump separate from left testicle.
(b) Epididymal cyst or spermatocele.
(c) Not unless it is giving discomfort or embarrassment to the patient.

85 (a) Urethral stricture — astride injury.
(b) Usually a short, tight stricture — by contrast, inflammatory (i.e. gonococcal) strictures may be long and ragged.
(c) Rough instrumentation of the urethra by an inexperienced surgeon: occasionally 'catheter' stricture after cardiac bypass surgery.

86, 87 (a) Teratoma of testis.
(b) Cord must be clamped at the internal ring before the testis is delivered and inspected; this prevents potential spread of tumour emboli.
(c) Alpha-feto protein (AFP) and human chorionic gonadotrophin (HCG) are commonly elevated in non-seminomatous germ cell tumours.
(d) No — gynaecomastia is usually observed in the rare sertoli cell tumour.

88 (a) Micturating cysto-urethrogram.
(b) Urethral stricture — post-bulbar. Bladder neck hypertrophy.
(c) Work hypertrophy as part of the detrusor effort to void.
(d) Treatment for stricture only — bladder neck *not* to be incised or resected despite appearances — may compromise continence if later surgical procedures are required at the level of the external urethral sphincter.

89, 90 (a) 'Hot spot' rib cage on bone scan (**89**).
(b) Tumour; injury (fracture); arthritis.
(c) Plain X-ray — showed that this lesion was due to a healing fracture. 'Hot spot' disappeared 12 months later (**90**).

91 (a) There is a calcified space-occupying lesion related to the lateral aspect of the left kidney.
(b) A simple renal cyst, 3% of which show calcification.
(c) A malignant tumour or alternatively a hydatid cyst.

92 (a) A percutaneous nephrostomy tube, placed to relieve obstruction and infection.
(b) Lithotripsy — the calculus shows fragmentation and passage of the calcific sand down the ureter.
(c) 12–14 days.

93, 94 (a) Urethral valves — endoscopic view and micturating cystogram.
(b) Pre-stenotic dilatation; severe bladder neck (work) hypertrophy; grossly trabeculated bladder and no reflux.
(c) Hydronephrosis, renal failure (if reflux not present, as illustrated, obstruction is present at the vesico-ureteric junction due to detrusor hypertrophy).
(d) Endoscopic destruction of valves with a bugbee catheter.

95–97 (a) Hypernephroma; rare skin lesions and common lytic bone disease.
(b) Nodal and intravascular (venous) tumour emboli.
(c) Left-sided varicocoele (obliterates the left testicular vein which joins the left renal vein).
(d) Highly unpredictable — patients with metastases often die within months but patients with apparently local tumours may live for many years after removal.

98, 99 (a) Transitional cell carcinoma of the lower ureter.

(b) Hydroureter; hydronephrosis.

(c) Excision of the lower ureter with reimplantation if the upper tract is disease free.

(d) Good — tumour is well organized with stalk formation.

100 (a) Pelviureteric junction obstruction.

(b) The kidney has taken 4 h to opacify; the ureter is seen in the upper third.

(c) Diuretic renogram.

(d) Distension pain, then acute relief as a large volume of urine is passed.

101 (a) Bladder diverticulum.

(b) Infection; stone formation; tumour (stasis).

(c) Micturating cystogram.

(d) Ureter.

102 (a) Hypernephroma.

(b) Glycogen and lipid within cytoplasm.

(c) Adenomata may be associated with the main tumour.

(d) None — hypernephroma was mistakenly so described by von Grawitz as both tumour and suprarenal are macroscopically yellow in appearance.

103 (a) Elick evacuator.

(b) Used for removing debris, blood clot or prostate chips from the bladder.

(c) Rupture of the bladder if an over-vigorous squeeze of the bulb occurs — particularly if the bladder wall has been weakened, for example, by tumour resection.

104–106 (a) The sessile hydatid of the testis is larger on one side, whilst the pedunculated hydatid (morgagni) of the epididymis is larger on the other. The sessile hydatid can be clearly seen if the scrotal wall is tensed.

(b) Torsion — usually of the pedunculated hydatid.

(c) Torsion of the testis.

(d) Para-mesonephric duct remnant.

107 (a) Bilateral upper tract filling defects — presume transitional cell tumour.
(b) Open local removal; percutaneous removal; uretero-resectoscopic removal (suitable for small tumour only).
(c) Ureteroscopy to assess further the possibility of multifocal disease within the upper tracts.

108 (a) Urethral condylomata.
(b) Blood spotting on underclothes.
(c) If multiple and/or within the urethra, electrocoagulation.
(d) Urethral stenosis if overzealous use of cautery.

109, 110 (a) Resectoscope — loop illustrated.
(b) 24 and 27 FG (French gauge).
(c) Urethral dilatation or otis urethrotomy.
(d) Urethral stricture.

111 (a) Inflow cystometrogram.
(b) Cough induced (three coughs shown) bladder instability.
(c) *Urge* incontinence of urine.
(d) Anticholinergic medication, e.g., imipramine at night.

112 (a) A space occupying lesion which contains gas, within the left kidney.
(b) A renal abscess.
(c) Surgical drainage or nephrectomy covered by appropriate antibiotic therapy.

113 (a) An antegrade pyelogram; percutaneous puncture of the pelvicalyceal system using a fine needle with contrast injection.
(b) A well-defined rounded filling defect within the pelvis, due to a lucent calculus.
(c) CT scanning — most apparently lucent calculi show a calcific rim when assessed by this technique.

114, 115 (a) Distortion of the pelvicalyceal systems of the large kidneys by multiple cysts.
(b) Adult-type polycystic disease, presenting in infancy. The ultrasound scan of infantile polycystic disease shows large echogenic kidneys, as the cysts are small (1 mm), causing reflection of sound from the multiple interfaces.

116, 117 (a) The typical tense (uterine-like) distended bladder of patients with high-pressure chronic retention.
(b) They demonstrate raised intravesical pressure — urine has risen up the tube. This does not happen within the normal bladder.
(c) Pressure is present throughout the fill–void bladder cycle and is responsible for development of hydronephrosis.
(d) Brisk haematuria (24–48 h) due to decompression.

118 (a) Intraperitoneal rupture of the bladder.
(b) As increasing peritonism (allow for other major injuries).
(c) Cystogram — dye has extravasated following injection into the bladder.
(d) Compression injury with a full bladder (often steering wheel impact).

119 (a) Transitional cell carcinoma of bladder.
(b) Haematuria.
(c) Deep resection biopsy to include muscle for histological assessment.
(d) Regular review cystoscopies for at least 10 years.

120, 121 (a) Renal pelvic stone; percutaneous nephrostomy in place.
(b) Percutaneous removal of the stone using lithotripsy (fragments illustrated).
(c) Septicaemia is a common and often life-threatening if infection is present during percutaneous surgery.

122 (a) Calcified lesion within the bladder.
(b) Calcified healing reaction following X-ray therapy.
(c) Resection and biopsy from the base to ensure that active disease is no longer present.

123 (a) Diathermy burn under plate electrode.
(b) Correct apposition of diathermy pad.
(c) Poor cutting or coagulation during the procedure — inadequate electrical circuit.

124 (a) The bladder wall.
(b) Urinary schistosomiasis.
(c) Ureteric strictures with subsequent ureteric obstruction and renal failure. There is also an increased risk of bladder neoplasm (squamous cell).

125(a) Retroperitoneal fibrosis. Intermittent abdominal or renal pain with progression to uraemia; raised erythrocyte sedimentation rate (ESR).
(b) Both pelvicalyceal systems are dilated and there is a band of abnormal tissue surrounding the aorta, inferior vena cava and ureters.
(c) Percutaneous nephrostomy to relieve obstruction and renal failure.
(d) Ureterolysis with omental wrapping.

126 (a) T1 tumours invade the lamina propria but do not reach muscle.
(b) On pathological examination the lesion is still found to conform to the definition above.
(c) Resection biopsy (to include muscle) for full pathological assessment.
(d) Hydronephrosis in a case of bladder tumour usually means muscle invasion is present, even if this is not seen endoscopically.

127 (a) Calcification of the right kidney and upper ureter.
(b) Tuberculous autonephrectomy: the advanced infection has destroyed the kidney and the ureter has been blocked by inflammatory debris. In these circumstances spontaneous sterilization of the infection can occur, with fibrosis and calcification.
(c) Healed tuberculosis of the spine at L2–3.

128, 129 (a) Amplatz dilators and sheaths for percutaneous surgery.
(b) Guide wire has been passed, percutaneous track dilated and sheath is in place prior to PCNL (percutaneous nephrolithotomy).
(c) Introduction of a nephroscope and shock wave treatment with aspiration of fragments.
(d) Percutaneous puncture could be performed under local anaesthetic, but dilatation of a 30FG sheath is uncomfortable and will require general or spinal anaesthesia.

130 (a) Mesonephric duct.
(b) Complete duplex ureter.
(c) The upper moiety ureteric orifice always inserts lower and more medially than the lower moiety ureteric orifice.
(d) Reflux caused by more direct path through the bladder wall.
(e) Ectopic opening of the upper moiety ureteric orifice, i.e. below the sphincters; into vaginal vault.

131, 132 (a) Incisional hernia.
(b) Usually ischaemic damage to at least two neurovascular bundles.
(c) Chronic cough, post-operative wound infection.
(d) Repair is rarely successful; support corset is often adequate.

133 (a) Urethral stricture — not particularly tight.

(b) A 'flat-topped' trace — often prolonged — is typical of urethral constriction.

(c) No — strictures are notoriously prone to recur.

(d) Uroflowmetry is required at each visit to judge objectively the progress of re-stenosis.

134 (a) Right-sided bladder tumour — likely to be transitional cell carcinoma. Left hydronephrosis and/or hydroureter.

(b) Hydronephrosis suggests multifocal disease may be present.

(c) Cystoscopy; left ureteroscopy or retrograde ureterogram to outline exactly any pathology in the left upper tract.

(d) Transurethral resection of the bladder lesion, including muscle, to assess the pathological stage and grade.

135 (a) Massive hydronephrosis; the pelvis shown contained 4.5 litres urine.

(b) Congenital pelvi-ureteric junction obstruction.

(c) Ache in the flank; intestinal compression symptoms.

136 (a) Prostate cancer (suggested by sudden onset of outflow tract symptoms).

(b) Acid, alkaline phosphatase.

(c) Chest X-ray; bone scan; plain X-rays of any 'hot spots'.

(d) Radiotherapy to the local deposit.

137 (a) Urethrogram — ascending.

(b) Post-bulbar stricture.

(c) Inflammatory aetiology — possible gonococcal infection.

(d) Internal urethrotomy.

138 (a) Multifocal transitional cell carcinoma.

(b) Smoking; dye workers; rubber workers: phenacitin abuse.

(c) Dyes used for colouring fish bait are highly carcinogenic.

139, 140 (a) Sachse urethrotomy knife.

(b) Incision of an urethral stricture.

(c) 12 o'clock within the urethra.

(d) Oedema and bruising beneath the penile and scrotal skin due to extravasation of irrigating fluid and blood.

141 (a) Urethral stone.
(b) Phimosis has prevented passage.
(c) Circumcision.

142, 143 (a) Isotope renogram — pictures from gamma camera.
(b) Hold-up in the kidneys and hydro-ureter, which resolves after the bladder has emptied.
(c) Reflux or vesico-ureteric obstruction due to bladder wall hypertrophy, as found in 'high pressure' retention or neurogenic bladder disorders.

144 (a) Obstruction to the venous return left leg (phlegmasia cærulea dolens).
(b) Malignant mass or nodal blockage of iliac veins.
(c) Very poor — high grade tumour of the upper tract carries limited prognosis.

145 (a) There is extravasation of intravenous contrast into the perinephric space.
(b) Acute loin pain, possibly with pyrexia.
(c) Obstruction of the upper ureter by a calculus (extravasation may also be precipitated by the osmotic diuretic effect of the contrast medium).

146 (a) Epididymal cysts.
(b) Palpable mass or 'dragging' sensation.
(c) Testis can be felt separately from the swelling (contrast hydrocele).
(d) Clear fluid (hydrocele — straw coloured fluid).

147, 148 (a) Sclerotic metastases in the bone.
(b) Raised acid, alkaline phosphatase.
(c) Prostate.
(d) Paget's disease in the right hemi-pelvis — coarse trabecular pattern and expansion of the bone are typical of this condition. Raised alkaline phosphatase is seen in both metastatic prostate cancer and Paget's, although the levels are usually very high in the latter condition.

149 (a) Transitional cell carcinoma of the ureter.
(b) Hydronephrosis.
(c) Poor barrier provided by a thin ureteric muscle (contrast bladder).
(d) Cuff of the bladder — total ureterectomy is required to prevent recurrence.

150, 151 (a) Replacement of the ureter by a small bowel; nephrostomy *in situ*.

(b) Irreversibly diseased ureter — such as may occur in tuberculosis.

(c) Absorption of urinary electrolytes.

(d) Passage of mucus in the urine.

152, 153 (a) Staghorn calculus (X-ray after removal).

(b) Infection; pyonephrosis.

(c) Loin pain; recurrent infection; septicaemia.

154 (a) Psoas abscess. Calcification of the wall of the aorta.

(b) Residual infected stone; suture material.

(c) Surgical drainage.

(d) Frequent recurrence at intervals.

155 (a) Very thick-walled bladder.

(b) Bladder neck obstruction.

(c) Urine flow test.

(d) Bilateral hydronephrosis may develop due to vesico-ureteric obstruction.

156 (a) Reflux cystogram.

(b) Grade III reflux filling the entire upper tract.

(c) Rarely — adequate fluid intake and antibiotics are the mainstay of treatment.

(d) Infection; reflux pyelonephritis; back ache (usually treated by antibiotics).

157 (a) Cyclophosphamide cystitis is characteristically bright red in appearance, following administration.

(b) Haemorrhagic cystitis.

(c) Alopecia; nausea; marrow depression.

158 (a) Bilateral 'cobra' heads, due to simple ureteroceles.
(b) The congenital cystic dilatation of the lower end of the ureter, when filled with intravenous contrast, produces an elliptical area of increased density within the bladder, surrounded by a radiolucent halo of the wall of the ureterocele.
(c) Few symptoms are to be expected from small 'simple' ureteroceles — hence these are often found in young adults.
(d) Approximately 10%.

159, 160 (a) Bladder stone.
(b) Strangury — pain from the trigone referred to the urethra.
(c) Removal *and* treatment of bladder outflow tract obstruction.

161, 162 (a) The double J stent, put in place for drainage of the kidney during lithotripsy, has become calcified *in situ*.
(b) Insertion of a percutaneous nephrostomy tube, followed by dissolution therapy.
(c) Endoscopically, using a flexible cystoscope under local anaesthesia.

163 (a) Bladder wall trabeculation increases as the bladder fills — emphasizing the subjective nature of this sign.
(b) Detrusor muscle bundles with collagen fibres.
(c) Muscle degenerates, collagen accumulates, leading to contractile dysfunction.

164 (a) Calcification and/or stones in the megalo-ureter.
(b) Congenital megalo-ureter.
(c) Reflux cystogram; antegrade pressure perfusion test (Whitaker test, to identify the obstruction).
(d) The area of interest for computer analysis must include the ureter.

165 (a) Prostatic 'chip' left in bladder at operation; now calcified.
(b) Urinary tract infection (UTI), dysuria or haematuria.
(c) Patients with a large 'floppy' decompensated bladder — the TUR chips are sometimes difficult to find and extract at operation.

166, 167 (a) Gross muscle hypertrophy, diverticula formation and trabeculation.
(b) Neurogenic (reflex bladder) disorder or high-pressure chronic retention.
(c) Obstruction at the vesico-ureteric junction.

168 (a) A persistent nephrogram with dilatation of the pelvicalyceal system on the left.
(b) The ureter is obstructed.
(c) Calculi, intrinsic ureteric tumours, extrinsic compression by malignant lymph nodes or distal stricture.

169 (a) Transitional cell carcinoma of the urethra.
(b) By careful urethroscopy with a 30° or 0° telescope; never instrument the urethra blindly in a case of suspected TCC urothelium.
(c) Strongly suggests the presence of multifocal disease.
(d) If cystectomy is considered, a urethrectomy must be performed at the same time.

170 (a) High-pressure chronic retention (large bladder, bilateral hydro-ureter and/or hydronephrosis).
(b) Late onset enuresis; reversible hypertension (pressure falls after catheter drainage); painless retention.
(c) Bladder outflow tract surgery resolves the upper tract signs.
(d) Gradually increasing uraemia leading to death.

171 (a) Ileal loop diversion.
(b) Hyperchloraemic acidosis may occur, particularly if renal function is impaired due to a previous pathological process.
(c) Invasive bladder cancer — cysto-urethrectomy.
(d) Appendicectomy.

172, 173 (a) Voiding cystometrograms — pressure/flow studies of bladder function.
(b) To enable subtraction of non-bladder pressures, such as cough, movement, etc., thus revealing the true detrusor pressure.
(c) **172**, high pressure, low flow (obstructed) voiding; **173**, low pressure, low flow voiding (underactive bladder dysfunction).

174, 175 (a) Filariasis.
(b) Wuchereria bancrofti.
(c) Eosinophilia.
(d) Surgery.
(e) Dimethylcarbamazine (maybe toxic, caution required).

176–178 (a) Thermometer and watch (illustrated) within the bladder.
(b) Strangury and recurrent infection.
(c) Patients often referred from mental institutions.
(d) Plain X-ray is always advisable however far-fetched the history may seem.

179, 180 (a) Torsion of testis — necrotic. Removal necessary.
(b) During the night and/or periods of rest. Not during activity.
(c) Transient pains, indicating twist episodes that resolved spontaneously.
(d) Other testicle *must* be fixed at the time of operation.

181 (a) Cystogram showing multiple diverticula.
(b) Severe urethral stenosis — rare in females; this resulted from obstetric trauma due to forceps delivery.
(c) Upper tract dilatation from vesico-ureteric obstruction.
(d) Regular (self) dilatation with bougie.

182–184 (a) Ovarian cyst — serous cystadenoma.
(b) Compression symptoms on the urogenital tract — patient presented in acute retention due to distortion of bladder from the cyst wedged in front of the sacrum.
(c) Ureter runs in the base of the pedicle.
(d) Must be removed intact to prevent fluid contamination within the peritoneum.

185, 186 (a) Squamous cell carcinoma of prepuce — base of the lesion has ulcerated through above the normal preputial opening.
(b) Infection; dysuria; bloody discharge.
(c) Antibiotic therapy should be instituted before assessing lymphatic spread — enlargement may be due to inflammation or neoplasia.
(d) Radiation or partial amputation if the growth involves the shaft or corpora cavernosa.
(e) Urethral stenosis after partial amputation.

187 (a) Bladder with diverticulum.

(b) Calcified lesion within the wall of the diverticulum.

(c) Stone (unlikely) or calcified tumour (probably).

(d) Poor if tumour — no muscle barrier in the wall of the diverticulum.

188 (a) Massive lymphadenopathy.

(b) Uraemia — ureteric compression.

(c) It is usually positive but a small number of patients may not have skeletal disease despite massive nodes.

(d) The large nodes are frequently highly hormone-sensitive, leading to prolonged survival.

189 (a) Normal trace.

(b) Typical obstructed trace.

(c) Flat trace of urethral stricture.

(d) Irregular trace, peak near mid-point — underactive bladder.

(e) Underactive bladder — urodynamics required to separate from (b).

(f) Intermittent flow rate — pushing to void or other abnormal habit.

190 (a) Verumontanum with overhanging right and smaller left lobe prostate.

(b) No — severe symptoms may be caused by small 'tight' prostates, yet few symptoms may result from large 100 g or more glands.

(c) Resection below the verumontanum may compromise the urethral sphincter function.

(d) Retrograde ejaculation is inevitable.

191, 192 (a) Micturating cystogram.

(b) Bilateral bladder diverticula — not emptying on micturition.

(c) 'Double micturition' — bladder refills from the diverticula and the patient experiences further desire to micturate.

(d) Excision of diverticula *and* treatment for bladder outflow obstruction.

193 (a) 'Micturating cystogram' in a young child, usually performed under general anaesthetic.
(b) The wooden spoon compresses the bladder to mimic micturition and demonstrate outlet obstruction or reflux.
(c) To protect the surgeon's hands from irradiation.
(d) It is rather unphysiological during the relaxation of general anaesthesia.

194, 195 (a) Swelling of testis and cord up into the abdomen.
(b) Lymphoma of testis — commonest testicular neoplasm in the elderly.
(c) Chest X-ray; IVP and CT abdomen to assess the disease extent.
(d) Despite treatment, poor with such rapid and massive growth.

Index

Numbers refer to the number shared by the illustration question and answer

Adenocarcinoma, 9, 10, 63, 64
Amplatz dilators and sheaths, 128, 129
Aorta wall calcification, 154
Appendicectomy, 171
Artificial sphincter, silicone pump, 28
[198]Au, 82

Balanitis xerotica obliterans, 17, 18
Ball diathermy electrode, 66, 67
Biopsy needle, 42
Bladder
  adenocarcinoma, 9, 10
  calcification of wall, 124
  calcified lesion, 122
  contractile dysfunction, 163
  distortion from ovarian cyst, 182–184
  diverticulum, 13, 101, 187, 191, 192
  Elick evacuator use, 103
  fill–void cycle, 116, 117
  fir-tree, 62
  foreign body in, 176–178
  function studies, 172, 173
  high-pressure chronic urine retention, 116, 117, 142, 143, 166, 167, 170
  instability, 111
  intraperitoneal rupture, 118
  low-pressure chronic retention, 14
  neck hypertrophy, 93, 94
  neck obstruction, 60, 61, 155
  neurogenic disorders, 62, 142, 143, 166, 167
  obstruction uroflow rate, 189
  outflow tract obstruction removal, 159, 160
  pre-stenotic dilatation, 93, 94
  prostatic chip, 165
  radical excisional surgery, 9, 10
  radiotherapy for cancer, 122
  reduction operation, 14
  space occupying lesion, 60, 61
  squamous cell carcinoma, 47
  stone, 13, 47, 159, 160, 187
  transitional cell carcinoma, 119, 134
  transurethral resection of lesions, 66, 67
  tumour, 82, 126, 134, 171, 187
  wall, 142, 143, 163, 166, 167
Bone scan, 53, 89, 90, 188
Bougie dilatation, 181
Bowel obstruction and strangulation, 48

Catheters, 77, 93, 94
Charrière gauge, 77
Chicken pox, 7
Chlamydia trachomatis, 54
Circumcision, 17, 18, 41, 141
Clear cell carcinoma of kidney, 63, 64
Coil embolization, 45, 46
Computed tomography (CT) scan, 56, 57, 69, 112, 187
Congenital abnormalities, 20, 21, 39, 40, 49, 50
Congenital megalo-ureter, 164
Congenital pelviureteric junction obstruction, 3, 4, 135
Corpus cavernosum, 75, 76
Coudé catheter, 77
Cryptorchidism, 69, 73
Cyclophosphamide cystitis, 157
Cystadenoma, serous, 182–184
Cystectomy, 169

Cystitis, haemorrhagic, 157
Cystogram
  intraperitoneal rupture of
      bladder, 118
  reflux, 156, 164
Cystogram, micturating, 191, 192,
    193
  bladder diverticulum, 101
  in pyelonephritis, 80
  urethral valves, 93, 94
Cystometrogram, 111, 172, 173
Cystoscopy, 15, 16, 134
Cystourethrectomy, 171
Cystourethrogram, micturating,
    62, 88

Diathermy burn, 123
Dietl's crisis, 100
Dimethylcarbamazine, 174, 175
Dormia basket, 43, 44
Double J stent, 161, 162
Drainage catheters, 77
Dysuria, 165

Ejaculation, retrograde, 190
Electrocoagulation of bleeding
    vessels, 66, 67
Elick evacuator, 103
Enuresis, late onset, 170
Epididymis
  cyst, 84, 146
  pedunculated hydatid, 104–106
Epididymitis, chronic discharging,
    48
Erythroplasia of Queyrat, *see*
    Paget's disease of penis

α-Feto protein, 86, 87
Filariasis, 174, 175
Fish bait dyes, 138

Gall bladder calculi, 26
Gil-Vernet incision, 22

Glans dislocation, 29
Gynaecomastia, 52, 86, 87

Haematuria
  bilateral staghorn calculi, 83
  congenital pelviureteric junction
      obstruction, 3, 4
  high-pressure chronic retention,
      116, 117
  hypernephroma, 95–97
  left hydronephrosis, 15, 16
  polycystic disease, 11, 12
  prostatic chip in bladder, 165
  transitional cell carcinoma, 119,
      149
Hemi-scrotum, 48, 69
Herpes zoster lesion, 7
Horseshoe kidney, 1, 2
Human chorionic gonadotrophin,
    86, 87
Hydatid cyst, calcified space-
    occupying lesion, 91
Hydrocele, 24, 25, 146
Hydronephrosis, 15, 16
  bladder tumour, 126
  congenital pelvi-ureteric
      junction obstruction, 135
  Dormia basket use, 43, 44
  fir-tree bladder, 62
  high-pressure urine retention,
      170
  percutaneous nephrostomy, 33
  prune belly syndrome, 73
  right-sided bladder tumour, 134
  transitional cell carcinoma of
      ureter, 98, 99
  ultrasound scan, 31
  ureterocele, 60, 61
  urethral valves, 93, 94
  vesico-ureteric obstruction, 155
Hydroureter, 98, 99, 134, 170
Hypernephroma, 5, 36–38, 45, 46,
    63, 64, 102
  adenomata associated with, 102
  haematuria, 95–97
  metastases, 56, 57, 68

prognosis, 95–97
Hyponatraemia, 66, 67

Ileal loop diversion, 171
Iliac fossa pain, 39, 40
Impotence, diabetes-related, 75, 76
Incisional hernia, 131, 132
Incontinence
    complete duplex ureter, 130
    squamous cell carcinoma of
        scrotum, 6
    surgery, 28
    urge, 111
Inferior vena cava, 56, 57
Inguinal lymph node examination,
    32
Isotope renogram, 27, 142, 143
IVU examination, 1, 2, 145

Jaboulay procedure, 24, 25

Kidney
    abnormal circulation pattern,
        36–38
    abscess, 112
    adenocarcinoma, 63, 64
    adenomata, 36–38, 102
    calcification, 127
    calcified space-occupying lesion,
        91
    calculi, 26
    clear cell carcinoma, 63, 64
    crossed ectopic, 39, 40
    cysts, 35, 91, 114, 115
    left hydronephrosis, 15, 16
    medullary pyramid tubule
        ectasia, 49, 50
    medullary sponge, 49, 50
    obstruction, 78, 79
    reflux, 156
    transitional cell carcinoma, 15,
        16
    tumour, 35, 45, 46, 70–72, 91
    ultrasound scan, 30, 31

Lithotripsy
    bilateral staghorn calculi, 83
    calcification of drainage stent,
        161, 162
    renal pelvic stone removal, 120,
        121
    for ureteric calculus, 92
Lithotriptor, 26
Loin incision, 22, 51
Lord procedure, 24, 25
Lucent calculus, 113
Lumbotomy approach, 22
Lymphadenopathy, massive in
    prostate, 188

Marion's sign, 23
Megalo-ureter calcification, 164
Mesonephric duct, 130
Micturition, double, 191, 192
Multifocal transitional cell
    carcinoma of ureter, 138

Nephrectomy, 36–38, 112, 154
Nephro-ureterectomy, 15, 16, 144
Nephroblastoma, see Wilm's
    tumour
Nephrocalcinosis, 49, 50
Nephrogram, persistent, 168
Nephrolithotomy, percutaneous,
    128, 129
Nephrostomy, 33, 92, 125, 150, 151
Nocturia, 55

Oestrogen therapy, 52
Orchidectomy, 48, 53
[123]Ortho-iodohippurate (OIH), 27
Otis urethrotomy, 109, 110
Ovarian cyst, 182–184
Oxalate calculus, 13

Paget's disease, 32, 147, 148
Papaverine self-injection, 75, 76
Para-mesonephric duct remnant,
    104–106

Paraphimosis, 41
Paraplegia, 29
Patent processus vaginalis, 24, 25
Pawnbroker sign, 84
Pelvic calculi removal, 22
Pelvic kidney, 20, 21
Pelvicalyceal system, 11, 12, 30, 31
Pelviureteric junction obstruction, 3, 4, 100
Penile prosthesis, 75, 76
Penis
  carcinoma, 32
  glans dislocation, 29
  Paget's disease, 32
  pressure necrosis, 29
Perineum, traumatic haemorrhage, 74
Phimosis, 102, 141
Phlegmasia caerulea dolens, 144
Polycystic disease, 11, 12, 114, 115
Polyuria, 55
Pre-stenotic dilatation of bladder, 93, 94
Prepuce, 41, 185–186
Prostate
  biopsy, 42
  diathermy burn, 123
  fluid pH, 54
  infection, 54
  massive lymphadenopathy, 188
  surgery, 23
  transurethral resection, 123
Prostate cancer, 136
  biopsy, 42
  bone scan, 89, 90
  gynaecomastia, 52
  hormonal manipulation, 53
  metastatic, 7
  radioisotope bone scan, 53
  sclerotic metastases in bone, 147, 148
  survival rate, 53
Prostatectomy, 23, 165
Proteus infection, 13
Prune belly syndrome, 73
Psoas abscess, 154
Pulmonary lobectomy, 68

Pulmonary metastases, cannon ball, 68
Pyelogram, antegrade, 113
Pyelonephritis, 20, 21, 80
Pyeloplasty, 3, 4
Pyonephrosis
  necrotic, 78, 79
  percutaneous drainage, 78, 79
  percutaneous nephrostomy, 33
  staghorn calculus, 152, 153
Pyuria, sterile, 81

Radiotherapy, 19, 52, 136
Reflux, Grade III, 156
Renal arteriogram, 45, 46
Renal cell carcinoma, 1, 2
Renal failure
  fir-tree bladder, 62
  left renal tumour with calcification, 71–72
  urethral valves, 93, 94
Renal impairment with bilateral staghorn calculi, 83
Renal incisions, 131, 132
Renal pelvic stone, 120, 121
Renal pelvis obstruction, 58, 59
Renogram, diuretic, 58, 59, 100
Resectoscope, 66, 67, 109, 110
Retroperitoneal fibrosis, 125

Sachse urethrotomy knife, 139, 140
Scarpa's fascia, 74
Schistosomiasis, 47, 124
Scrotum, 6, 74
Seminoma, 19, 68
Spermatocele, 84
Squamous cell carcinoma
  of bladder, 47
  of prepuce, 185–186
  of scrotum, 6
Staghorn calculus, 83, 152, 153
Staphylococcus aureus, 33
Stasis of contrast, 1, 2
Steinstrasse, 65
Stone formation, 1, 2, 3, 4
Strangury, 159, 160

Testis
hydatid structures, 104–106
lymphoma, 194, 195
pawnbroker sign, 84
seminoma, 19
swelling, 194, 195
teratoma, 86, 87
torsion, 104–106, 179, 180
tumour, 24, 25
Transitional cell carcinoma, 107
of bladder, 119
of kidney, 15, 16
of ureter, 98, 99, 149
of urethra, 169
Trucut biopsy needle, 42
Tuberculosis, 48, 81, 127, 150, 151
Tuberculous autonephrectomy, 127
TUR syndrome, 66, 67

Ultrasound scan, 26
of kidney, 30, 31, 34, 35, 36–38
of upper abdomen, 56, 57
Upper pole calyx stenosis, 81
Uraemia, 125
Ureter
calcification, 127
calculus, 92, 145
complete duplex, 130
excision with reimplantation, 98, 99
obstruction, 168
replacement by a small bowel, 150, 151
stone visualization, 26
transitional cell carcinoma, 98, 99, 107, 138, 144, 149
Ureteric strictures in urinary schistosomiasis, 124
Ureterocele, 60, 61, 158
Ureterogram, retrograde, 134
Ureterolysis, 125
Ureteroscopy, 107, 134

Urethra
blood and mucus, 9, 10
condylomata, 108
dilatation for resectoscope use, 109, 110
obstruction in balanitis xerotica obliterans, 17, 18
stone, 141
transitional cell carcinoma, 169
Urethral stenosis, 17, 18, 32, 108, 181, 185, 186
Urethral stricture, 85, 133
micturating cyst-urethrogram, 88
post-bulbar, 137
resectoscope complications, 109, 110
Sachse urethrotomy knife, 139, 140
uroflow rate, 189
Urethral valves, 93, 94
Urethrogram, ascending, 137
Urethroscopy, 169
Urethrotomy, 137
Urinary infection, 13, 14
Urine
frequency volume chart, 55
passage of mucus, 150, 151
retention, 170
see also Incontinence
Uroflow rates, 133, 189

Varicocoele, 95–97
Vascular occlusion by coil embolization, 45, 46
Verumontanum, 190
Vesico-ureteric junction obstruction, 166, 167
Voided bladder specimens, 54
Von Grawitz tumour, 63, 64

Wilm's tumour, 8
Wucheria bancrofti, 174, 175